HIGH
ENERGY
LIVING

The Prevention Total Health System®

HIGH ENERGY LIVING

by the Editors of
Prevention® Magazine

 Rodale Press, Emmaus, Pennsylvania

Printed in the United States of America on recycled paper containing a high percentage of de-inked fiber.

Library of Congress Cataloging in Publication Data
Main entry under title:

High energy living.

(The Prevention total health system)
On t.p. the registered trademark symbol "R" is superscript following "Prevention" in the statement of responsibility and following "system" in the series.
Includes index.
1. Health.   2. Vitality.
I. Prevention (Emmaus, Pa.) II. Series.
RA776.5.H44   1985   613   85-19606
ISBN 0-87857-554-5   hardcover
2 4 6 8 10 9 7 5 3 1   hardcover

NOTICE

The Prevention Total Health System®
Series Editors: William Gottlieb, Mark Bricklin
High Energy Living Editor: Debora Tkac
Writers: Mike McGrath (Chapters 1, 9), Camille Cusumano, Carol Keough (Chapter 2), Gerry Hunt (Chapter 3), Nicholas S. Yost (Chapter 4), Joseph N. Farrell (Chapter 5), Dary Matera (Chapters 6, 11), Bill Keough (Chapter 7), Nona Cleland (Chapters 8, 10).
Research Chief: Carol Baldwin
Associate Research Chief, Prevention Health Books: Susan Nastasee
Assistant Research Chief, Prevention Health Books: Holly Clemson
Researchers: Carole Rapp, Jill Jurgensen, Martin Wood, Jan Eickmeier, Martha Capwell, Lynda Pollack
Copy Editor: Jane Sherman
Copy Coordinator: Joann Williams
Series Art Director: Jane C. Knutila
Designers: Lynn Foulk, Alison Lee
Illustrators: Bascove, Susan Gray, Mary Anne Shea, Elwood Smith, Chris Spollen
Project Assistants: Lisa Gatti, Margot J. Weissman
Director of Photography: T. L. Gettings
Photo Editor: Margaret Skrovanek
Staff Photographers: Carl Doney, John Hamel, Margaret Skrovanek, Christie C. Tito
Photographic Stylists: Anne Hakanson, Renee R. Keith, J. C. Vera
Photo Researcher: Donna Lewis
Production Manager: Jacob V. Lichty
Production Coordinator: Barbara A. Herman
Composite Typesetter: Brenda J. Kline
Production Administrator: Eileen Bauder
Office Personnel: Susan K. Lagler, Roberta Mulliner, Janet Schuler

Rodale Books, Inc.
Publisher: Thomas Woll
Senior Managing Editor: William H. Hylton
Assistant Managing Editor: Ann Snyder
Art Director: Jerry O'Brien
Director of Marketing: Pat Corpora
Director of Book Production, Trade Sales and Subsidiary Rights: Ellen J. Greene

Rodale Press, Inc.
Chairman of the Board: Robert Rodale
President: Robert Teufel
Executive Vice President: Marshall Ackerman
Group Vice Presidents: Sanford Beldon
                                    Mark Bricklin
Senior Vice President: John Haberern
Vice Presidents: John Griffin
                         Richard M. Huttner
                         James C. McCullagh
                         David Widenmyer
Secretary: Anna Rodale

Contents

Preface

Energy Puts Quality in Living

If human energy were nothing more than mere get-up-and-go, then 4-year-olds would be more productive than 40-year-olds. Your kid would go out and work for you instead of the other way around.

But human energy—meaningful, purposeful energy—is a lot more than the raw force that makes boilers boil, flags flap, and four-year-olds irrepressible.

Human energy means getting your act together.

It's the chemical reaction between necessity and invention. Between desire and deed. Between putting your life on hold and exclaiming, "Hold everything!"

Human energy has different speeds. Life in the fast lane too often means nothing more than beating friends to the red light. Others may spend their life in the breakdown lane and dream, perhaps, of Mercedes Benz tow trucks.

My own favorite speed on the winding road of life is 45. You can take in the scenery, have a good sense of the road and get pretty near optimum fuel efficiency to boot. Cruising speed.

Whatever speed you choose to cruise, the real idea is to enjoy yourself. Getting there isn't half the fun, it's all there is.

Sometimes, though, momentum slips gears. We may knock and sputter. We may quit hoping for a valve job from heaven and start praying for a good firm shoulder. Maybe even one to cry on.

High Energy Living says it's all part of the trip. Repairing and regenerating your personal momentum from time to time is natural. There's not a single creative person I know who hasn't felt burned-out, lost, becalmed or dead in the water. Read the biographies of great people and you'll read of weeks or months of great confusion or depression or exhaustion. Somehow, they got themselves going again.

This is a book of "somehows." Hundreds of them. And one of them has a handle that's just right for your grip.

The solution may be to quit being a perfectionist. It may be to eat fewer sweets or more iron. To get more sleep or get up earlier in the morning. To drink less coffee or less wine. To build more self-confidence or lose weight. To do less long-distance running or less long-distance TV watching. To get the kids off your back and go back-packing in the mountains. To go to the doctor for a thorough checkup or write an outrageous check to your travel agent. Maybe both. Just knowing about these options is an energy booster.

Ultimately, you will learn that the best way to enjoy high-energy living is not to wait for a dead battery before you begin recharging yourself. Fun and games, music and meandering, should be part of your everyday agenda. A speedometer stuck at one speed is in a rut no matter what the number reads. Energy is the ability to change. To smell new ideas like beautiful flowers.

This volume of The Prevention Total Health System® is a meadow of fresh ideas.

Executive Editor, **Prevention**® Magazine

1

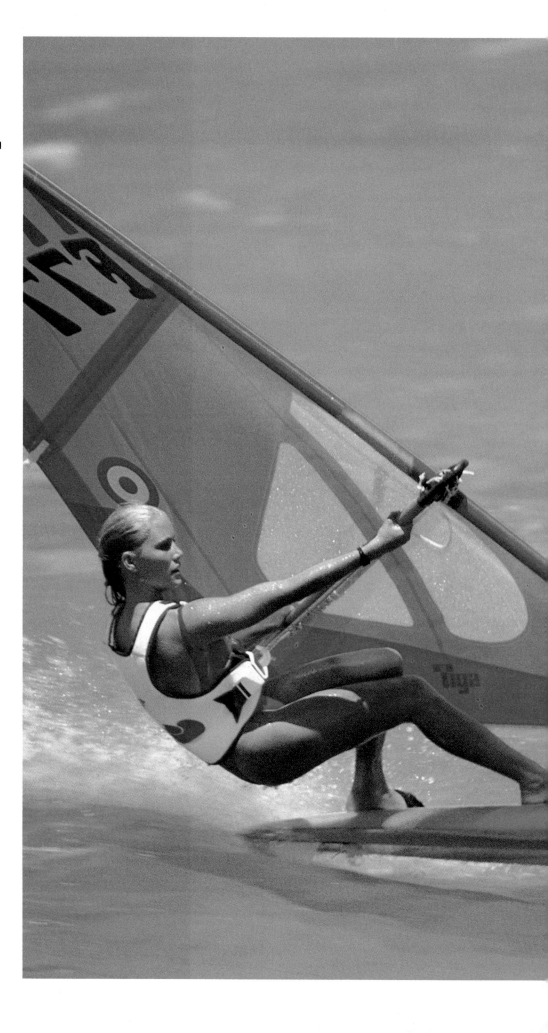

Energy— What a Wonderful Feeling!

Personal energy comes in many guises. Get them all in peak form and you're on your way to a turbocharged life.

It was the most important scientific discovery of the century, maybe of all time, and it was summed up in one, short formula that's now as familiar to us as our own names: $E=mc^2$. The E, of course, stands for energy, and the equation means that *everything* in the universe is a form of energy, sculptures made out of captured light.

Well, adjust a few letters and numbers, and the formula is true of us, too: $E=me$. Because everything "me" is—everything you are and do—is a form of energy.

Is your body strong and flexible, ready to tackle just about any job, from putting out the garbage to putting up this season's (huge!) tomato crop? If it is, you've got *physical* energy. If it isn't, you probably feel about as lively as a throw pillow.

Feeling good about yourself and others? *Emotional* energy is 150 watts and shining. Or does your world seem as bright as the bottom of a trash bin? Somebody turned out the lights.

Have you read a book in the last month or so that really made you think—maybe even changed your opinions about a subject? Or is your mind as closed as a window in January? Thinking in new ways (a must for creativity and problem solving) is one sign of *mental* energy.

Do you ever set long-term goals for your life? Or rededicate yourself to a cherished ideal, whether it's being more helpful to your next-door neighbor or helping save children in a foreign land? If so, you've got *spiritual* energy. Without it, you can feel a little like a lost puppy—directionless and scared.

These four types of energy are like the four

1

sides of a foundation—the structure on which you can build a happy, healthy life. And this book is like a blueprint for that structure, a super-practical guide to an "energy-efficient" you. But for a minute or two we'd like to be a little *im*practical, and take you on a short tour through the cells of your own body. Because it's there—in a biochemical process that has the unrelenting precision of a megabyte computer and the stunning delicacy of a rose bush in bloom—that energy begins.

ATP: ENERGY'S MONOGRAM

We've all seen models of molecules, those stick-and-ball structures that look like they were built with Tinker Toys by a persistent three-year-old. Well, the ATP (shorthand for adenosine triphosphate) molecule was put together by a prodigy.

The "sticks" in most molecules—the bonds that connect the chemical "balls"—are about as energetic and changeable as fence posts. But some of the sticks in ATP are more like firecrackers. They can explode at any time. And when they do, they release huge amounts of energy—many times more than a normal chemical bond. For this reason, these links in ATP are called "high-energy phosphate" bonds. And there's something else special about ATP. When it creates energy, it releases a phosphate ion and becomes ADP (adenosine diphosphate). The phosphate ion, with the help of cellular nutrients, then combines with the ADP to form *more* ATP. That means ATP is the body's inexhaustible energy account, and scientists have dubbed it energy currency because it can be spent and remade again and again.

Where does all that energy go? ATP is the fuel of the cells. And cells are the powerhouses of the body. ATP moves blood sugar, sodium, calcium and lots of other in-demand substances in and out of the cells. ATP helps make nutrients and other chemicals. (When a single protein is formed, for instance, several *thousand* ATP molecules have to get into the act.) And ATP sparks muscle. Without it, no muscle in the body could contract—you couldn't be holding

this book or moving your eyes across the page.

In short, ATP is at the center of energy in the body. And sometimes it seems like a few people have more ATP—or more something—than the rest of us. These are the people who never seem to get tired, and sometimes you wonder if their achievements are simply calculated to make you look bad. After all, they work harder than you do and seem to play harder than you work.

STRESS: AN ENERGY BOOSTER

Could the difference be as simple as the way they handle the daily physical and mental pressure we call stress? William F. Fry, Jr., M.D., a California psychiatrist, reminds us that stress and pressure in our lives have been accused of causing every modern evil from heart attacks to halitosis. These negative pressures were called dystress by the late Hans Selye, M.D.

But, beginning in the 1970s, Dr. Selye—known as the father of stress theory—started to discuss the notion of the *positive* aspects of stress: certain types and amounts that actually contribute to better health. He called this type eustress (from the same Greek root as the word *euphoria*).

Dr. Fry feels that everyone can benefit from—in fact, needs—this kind of positive stress in their lives. We are "children of stress," he says, and it is only by reacting cleverly and ambitiously to the problems in our lives that we have grown and developed as a species. Being faced with vast distances to cross, for instance, didn't make us sick or distraught—it prodded us to build boats and bridges, to tame horses and finally to create horseless carriages, airplanes and space shuttles.

As we will see, the people we call stress seekers just naturally seem to be better at turning stress into eustress rather than dystress.

Suzanne Kobasa, Ph. D., teaches psychology at the graduate school of City University of New York. She describes people who manage to be both stressed and healthy as "hardy" individuals. Dr. Kobasa feels that this quality of "hardiness" allows

Your Body's Energy Network

Just where *does* your energy come from? What's actually happening inside your body when you feel a burst of creativity, when your senses and muscles suddenly "come alive," when you're excited or surprised? The process seems amazingly complex, yet it's actually very simple and straightforward. Your body's energy network is activated by these inner functions:

Brain

Energy begins in the brain, unless it's too tired. A lack of oxygen-rich blood can make our most important organ fatigued and unable to perform the way we'd like. In fact, the brain requires up to 30 times as much blood as other organs to fuel the nerve cells called neurons that transmit information by way of electrical impulses that cross the synapses from one neuron to another.

Reticular Formation

Inside the stem of the brain is a very complex network about the size of your little finger. The reticular formation is packed with millions of neurons that tell your brain when to be awake and when to sleep. In addition to actually keeping you alert and conscious, this network keeps your muscles in shape and helps control your physical movements.

Nervous System

There is one part of the nervous system that controls the functioning of the inner organs. It has two divisions. One (the parasympathetic) keeps you cool, calm and collected by reducing your blood pressure and heart rate; the other (the sympathetic) drives you into action—it pumps blood and speeds up your heart rate and metabolism to wake you up and fill you with energy.

Pituitary Gland

Just under the brain lies the "master gland"—the pituitary. It produces no less than six well-defined hormones. One of these, known as ACTH, stimulates the adrenal cortex, activating the release of the hormone cortisol. All this happens when you realize that something stressful or exciting is about to occur. You can feel the energy surge.

Thyroid Gland

Wrapped around the windpipe, the thyroid serves as the body's thermostat. The thyroid and its two associated glands, the pituitary and the hypothalamus, constantly exchange information that regulates the amount of thyroid hormone. This determines how the body's fuel is used up. Too much or too little hormone and the body's "engine" runs too fast or too slow.

Adrenal Glands

Located near the kidneys, the adrenal glands pump out adrenaline to energize you. The adrenaline, or epinephrine, produced by the adrenal glands during periods of stress prepares your body for instant action. The heart races, the liver releases stored blood sugar, and the blood pressure itself rises, forcing that sugar into the muscles and brain.

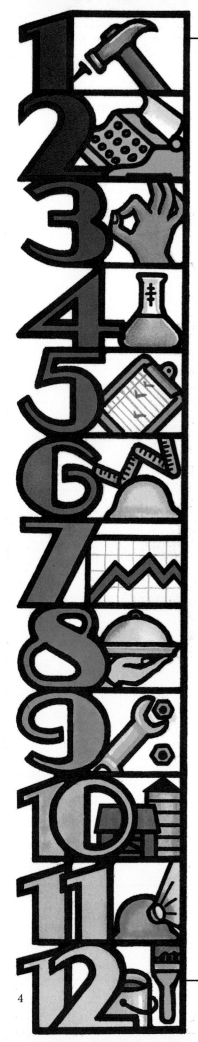

The 12 Most Stressful Jobs

Which jobs *really* cause the most stress?

To find out, the National Institute for Occupational Safety and Health (NIOSH) looked at hospital, mental health and death records to see which jobs actually made workers crazy, contributed to illness and even led to early death.

The results were surprising. Doctors, lawyers and other such "obvious" choices were conspicuously absent—their stress was offset by recognition and high pay. The following occupations were the ones found to be most hazardous to your well-being:

- Laborer
- Secretary
- Inspector
- Laboratory technician
- Office manager
- Foreman
- Administrator
- Waiter and waitress
- Machine operator
- Farm owner
- Mine worker
- Commercial painter

Just below this "top 12" was a cluster of occupations in the health care field (nurses, aides, technicians) and public service workers (police, firemen, social workers).

What do these overly stressed workers have in common? According to NIOSH, jobs with an unrelenting pace, boring work, lack of recognition and little or no control over the work situation.

some people to be subjected to a great number of stressful events in their work without being harmed by the experience. Indeed, as is obvious in some of our examples and in the energetic people around us, there are those who seem to positively *thrive* on the stress that makes others ill.

What characterizes a hardy person? To find the answer, Dr. Kobasa studied a large group of executives at Illinois Bell Telephone.

The executives who were able to cope positively with the stress of their work and personal lives exhibited three important characteristics not found among less hardy executives: commitment, control and challenge.

"People strong in *commitment*," Dr. Kobasa observes, "find it easy to be interested in whatever they are doing and can involve themselves in it wholeheartedly.

"People strong in *control*," she says, "believe and act as if they can influence the events taking place around them."

People strong in a sense of *challenge*, says Dr. Kobasa, "consider it natural for things to change and anticipate the changes as a useful stimulus to development."

The difference between dystress and eustress, between ennui and energy, may simply be in the way we *look* at events. High-energy people seem to have a different way of perceiving the world. Situations that frighten some people into a blind panic seem like an invigorating challenge to those who thrive on stress.

Maurice J. Martin, M.D., professor and chairman of psychiatry and psychology at Mayo Medical School in Minnesota, points out that *all* of us can learn to look at stress positively.

Perhaps that's what the people profiled in this chapter really have going for them. Like true stress seekers, they view life as a challenge, not as a threat. Whether or not they came into the world with extra energy, they lead the kind of lives that build and develop what they have. The famous trial lawyer Louis Nizer, now in his eighties, says this use of energy was present in every great achiever he had ever met, yet it was different in each: "Energy," he explains, "takes various forms and has as many facets as a good diamond."

Who Are the Stress Seekers?

Remember the Broadway show *What Makes Sammy Run?* Sammy, it seems was a stress seeker—one of those people who are not diminished by the stress in their life but actually thrive on it. For these individuals, too much is never enough; why walk when you can run?

Some experts feel that such people have a "biological need" for stimulation and seek it out, while others theorize that their energy is inherited. Whatever the case, here's a rundown on the top 10 characteristics that separate the stress seekers from the rest of us.

1 They're Committed to Self-Improvement.
Positive stress seekers are rarely satisfied with their own performance. The challenge to excel, to do better than ever, is like the force that drives athletes to break not only other people's records but their own as well.

2 They Tend to Procrastinate.
Those who thrive on stress often seem to find a way to create a stressful situation in order to do their best work. Putting things off till the last minute builds the pressure that helps them work better.

3 They Constantly Search for Challenge.
Stress seekers do not take the easy road very often, and this applies to their careers as well. Challenge or novelty is what they look for in a work environment —a chance to win every day.

4 They Face Problems Head-On.
People who function best under pressure are not put off by obstacles. What someone else might perceive as a stop sign is to them a challenge to their intellect, creativity and ability, something they must turn to their own advantage.

5 They Search for Energizing Activities.
Naturally, these people who welcome stress into their lives, homes and careers aren't going to leave it behind when it comes to leisure time. They work hard, play hard and often take the kind of vacations that would exhaust others.

6 They Like to Take Risks.
We're talking mountain climbing, survival camping and parachute jumping here. While not exactly reckless, these kinds of activities do attract people who like to meet life head-on. To them, the risk is worth the reward: excitement.

7 They Tend to Be Nonconformists.
A regular, suburban, middle-class lifestyle is not exactly appealing to true seekers of stress. Unstructured living seems to feed the creative impulses they need to look at the world in their decidedly different way.

8 They're People Who Need People.
No one can be creative in a vacuum, and the stress seekers, who want to be more creative than most, are no exception. They depend on the people around them to be sources of new ideas and stimulation.

9 They Get Bored Very Quickly.
One of the prices this breed of person has to pay for their unique outlook is an extremely low tolerance for activities that are repetitious, dull and boring. Without change and stimulation they can become restless and discontented.

10 They Thrive on Deadlines.
Since stress seekers live for pressure, it's only natural that to them, "the dreaded deadline doom" is just the opposite—another welcome challenge that gets those creative juices flowing.

High-Energy People

Who are some of the people who've gone for the gusto with great success? They come from totally different walks of life and use their energy in remarkably different ways. But all have one thing in common: a real passion for life and work that gives them the drive to carry on, to go that "extra mile" (or extra song, extra base, extra book . . .).

Bruce Springsteen

Previously a skinny, scrawny rock 'n' roller who had "never exercised before in my whole life," Bruce Springsteen pumped up with weight training and ran 6 miles a day to prepare for the rigors of his multiyear international "Born in the USA" tour. Not only did The Boss (as his fans call him) lose 3 to 5 pounds every night due to the intense aerobic acrobatics of his 3½- to 4-hour shows, he had started that day with the exact same performance! While other rockers would rush through or simply pass on a "sound check" of the hall, Springsteen would play through his *entire* set for the evening earlier in the day, have some dinner and then play it again "for real" that night. Where does he get the energy? Certainly not from drugs, which have no place in Springsteen's tour or his life. "I get the strength and the energy from the crowd," he explains.

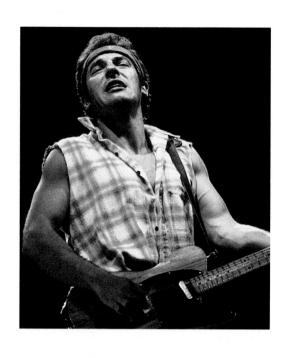

Louis Nizer

A legend in the legal world, this chief partner of one of New York's most prestigious law firms had just turned 83 the day before we spoke with him. The tremendous personal energy that had gained Louis Nizer a reputation for exhausting his younger associates was undiminished. "I'm working harder today than I did years ago," he says. "I just finished a 3-week trial and very often I would work here at the office with witnesses or with my associates on legal research till 3:00 or 4:00 in the morning; then I'd go to court at 9:00. Many times I'd just wash my face and go to court without going to sleep." Where does he find the time for other pursuits, like the paintings that win prizes, the music he composes, the books he writes (9 published so far), the speaking engagements?

"When I'm vacationing," he explains, "in addition to reading legal briefs, I paint. I find it relaxing. I brought back 6 paintings from my last trip."

Like others with high-energy lives, Nizer also feels that "I waste more time than most people I know. At night we'll go out socially for dinner and then play gin till 1:00 in the morning. I watch TV—I love to watch hours of sports. We all waste lots of time."

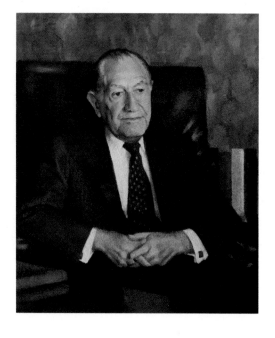

Joan Benoit Samuelson

What's so special about Joan Benoit Samuelson? Okay, so she shattered the world record by almost 3 full minutes in the 1983 Boston Marathon and then went on to a decisive gold-medal victory in the first women's marathon ever held at the Olympics. A lot of people run, right? But do they train for the Olympics while restoring a "shambles" of an 1853 house on Maine's unforgiving craggy coast? Do they finish 11-mile training runs with a nice, relaxing round of splitting logs for the fire—in January? Joan seems to spend much of her time looking not for extra energy but for extra energy outlets. "I don't cut workouts short very often," she told *Runner's World* magazine. Instead she adds a couple of miles. Probably to relax.

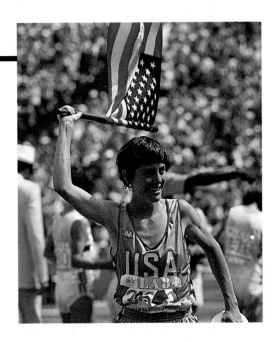

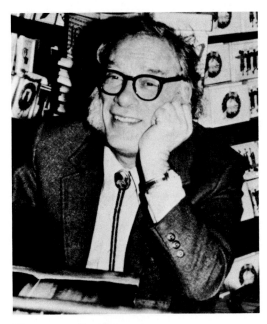

Isaac Asimov

This one-man operation—he answers his own phone and doesn't even have a typist—has had 212 books published in the 14½ years since he moved his office to New York City. That's about a book every 3 weeks, and it doesn't include the 100 or so he had written previously. "It's not the quantity I'm proud of," he says. "What strikes me as surprising is the wide variety of the type of work I do." The variety includes hard science, popular science, science fiction, history, biography, collections of "lecherous limericks," guides to Shakespeare and other literary criticism, mysteries, short stories and anthologies. His secret? "Writing is all I do; I'm at the typewriter at 7:30 A.M. and I stay there till 10:00 P.M."

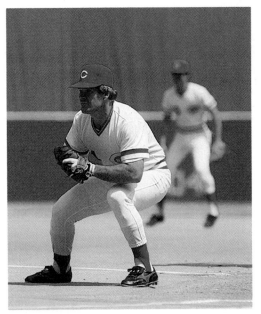

Pete Rose

Even way past his 40th birthday, the man with the most hits ever, plus the most singles, games played and times at bat in the National League still ran to first base when the pitcher walked him. And he could always be counted on to make the turn and try a head-first slide for home when almost any other ballplayer would stop at third. But no other ballplayer is quite like the man they call Charlie Hustle. "It's like he's in high gear all the time," says batting coach Billy DeMars. "The son of a gun never drops down to first gear; he's always in fourth." Says Rose of himself, "I didn't get to the majors on God-given ability—I got there on hustle, and I have had to hustle to stay."

Feats of Endurance and Strength

Ladies, gentlemen, children of all ages—step right up and witness with your very own eyes the most amazing feats of human strength and endurance ever presented within the limited confines of two pages. . . .

Man Lifts Over Three Tons

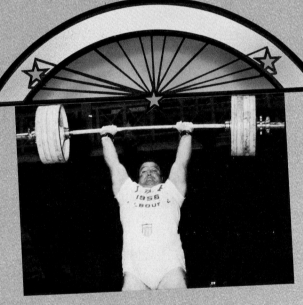

It's hard to imagine, but 1956 Olympic weight-lifting champion Paul Anderson managed to back-lift a table covered with auto parts and a safe full of lead off the trestles supporting it. That 6,270 pounds represents the greatest weight ever lifted by a human. Speaking of auto parts, we were also impressed to hear that Arthur Dandurand picked up a 455-pound automobile engine, carried it for 84 feet and then set it down on a table. Gently, we hope.

Nyad Swims 89 Miles Nonstop!

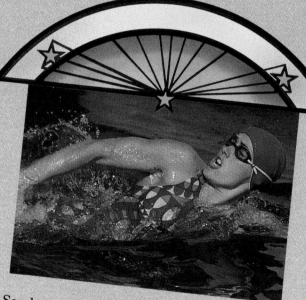

So who cares about the English Channel! It's *only* 21 miles across, and by 1981 over 200 people, including a 58-year-old, had swum across. Michael Reed crossed it 23 times and John Erikson spent over 38 hours in the water to complete the first *triple* crossing in 1981. But Diana Nyad broke *all* the distance records when she swam the open sea from Bimini to Florida—89 nautical miles in just 27 hours and 43 minutes. And she did it just two weeks after a previous attempt had been foiled when she was temporarily paralyzed by repeated stings from a deadly Portuguese man-of-war. She braved sharks and the currents of the Gulf Stream, and was "only" stung repeatedly by jellyfish this time. Why did the 30-year-old marathon swimmer, who had already crossed Lake Ontario and circumnavigated the island of Manhattan, attempt such a feat? "It all comes down to pride," she told *Newsweek*, "the satisfaction of overcoming something that seems impossible."

Pair Conquers Borneo

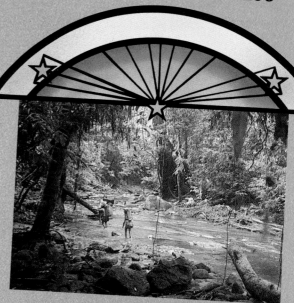

The Ultimate Athletes

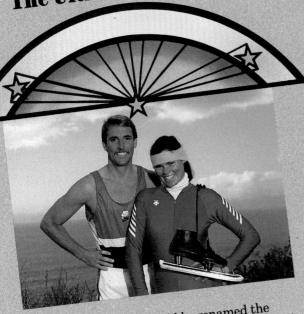

Maybe the triathlon should be renamed the die-athlon. To win the Ironman Triathlon competition in Hawaii, for instance, Californian Dave Scott had to swim 2.4 miles, bike another 112 across lava beds (often against 50-mile-per-hour headwinds), *then* run a full 26.2-mile marathon just as the temperature hit about 90°F, with 85 percent relative humidity.

Then there's top ski racer and mountaineer Jan Reynolds, who attempted the Mountain Man Triathlon in Colorado—described as "one of the most brutal tests of mountaineering and endurance that the body is capable of performing in one day"—with a bad sinus infection.

She did fine on the ski course that began 7,740 feet up the side of a mountain, went down a powder run, then continued back up to the 11,440-foot summit and back to the lodge for a total of 11 miles. She then put on snowshoes, climbed 2,000 feet up a hill, ran along a ridge and then back down the hill for a total of 8½ miles. But when she put on ice skates to do 28 laps (over 12 miles), her ankles gave out after 5 laps. Instead of quitting, though, she continued, skating in pain to finish in just under 6½ hours. Other triathletes were still coming in 1½ hours later.

In 1983, six noted outdoor athletes attempted the first-ever complete jungle crossing of the heavily forested tropical island of Borneo. Forty-three days later, the two who survived disease and disillusion (the others turned back) emerged on the eastern coast. But not before having endured a river ride that included 28 miles of suicidal rapids; a blazing equatorial sun; near-constant mud, thorns, wasps and leeches; and a trek through a slow-burning forest fire where temperatures reached 175 degrees and the adventurers had to walk across a 100-foot-long smoldering log where a misstep would pitch them into hot, glowing embers some 25 feet below. All this without ever being quite sure of where they were, since that unexplored portion of the jungle appears only as a huge blank spot on the government's topographic maps.

9

Energy Forever

Sixty. To many who have reached or are approaching that age in life, it can be a depressing number, more dreaded than the feared four-zero, the big half-century or the awesome double nickel. But to fitness fanatic and all-around high-energy ball of fire Jack LaLanne, 60 was a challenge.

For *his* 60th birthday, LaLanne wanted to prove he was getting better instead of older, so he decided to repeat a previous "impossible" accomplishment.

Nineteen years before, LaLanne had celebrated his 41st birthday with a swim from Alcatraz to San Francisco's Fisherman's Wharf.

Alcatraz—the inescapable prison. If you manage to reach the water, the treacherous currents that move constantly through the area are a veritable death sentence. LaLanne became the first to swim it successfully—*and* he was handcuffed!

Now he was 60. Time to slow down and take things easy. So he repeated the swim—handcuffed, with his feet shackled *and* while towing a 1,000-pound boat.

LaLanne was 62 during the Bicentennial; he celebrated by towing 13 boats that were carrying 76 people a mile across the harbor in Long Beach, California. It took him over an hour to pull the 25,000-pound load, and his pulse was a remarkably low (but patriotic) 76 shortly after.

Sixty-five. Retirement age, right? Jack retired by towing 65 boats carrying a total of 6,500 pounds of wood pulp for a mile across a lake near Japan's Mt. Fuji.

When he reached 70, he was finally ready to act his age. This time he towed 70 boats with 70 people aboard for a mile—handcuffed and shackled, of course.

We asked him why he wasn't satisfied with ice cream and cake like almost everybody else.

"I do these birthday feats just to prove to people, especially myself, that as you get older, you can still accomplish the things you had never been able to do in your life. Age is *just* a number.

"You know why there's so many screwed-up old people in this society? It's because they're put into pigeon-holes. After we're 'little kids' and 'teenagers,' we become 'middle-aged,' then we're 'senior citizens.'

" 'Middle-aged' people think, 'I'm going to have a heart attack. I'm losing my sex drive and my youth is going down the tubes'—and when they get to be 'senior citizens,' they picture Alzheimer's disease and people sitting around being fed, all crippled up with arthritis and rheumatism. It's these mental pictures that screw us up. I have friends who are 80 (and up) years old and they have more zip than I'll ever have!"

Physical fitness isn't the only defense against aging, and LaLanne

---

"Old" Is Just a Label

In 1983, the Kripalu Center for Yoga and Health in Lenox, Massachusetts, offered a week-long workshop titled "Retirement: Having the Time of Your Life," which their catalog described as "especially designed for people who choose to remain actively involved with life even though their occupational commitments are drawing to a close."

What the workshop organizers didn't realize was just *how* "actively involved with life" the attendees would become. It seems that, after a few days of stretching and a change in diet, "their energy picked up, their mental and physical barriers relaxed, and they discovered just how good their bodies could feel," explains Frances Mellen, program director.

Many of the participants felt *so* good, in fact, that they left the workshop "to get involved in all the 'normal' activities" at the center. The planners began to wonder if it had really been necessary to gear a workshop toward these "older people."

"The workshop *was* successful," Ms. Mellen explained, "but we also found out that retired people integrate extremely well into all our programs." It seems this was one weekend where *everyone* learned something.

points out that it doesn't have to be exercise that's the driving interest in your life—as long as you're interested in *something*.

"You have to be passionate," he says. "You have to enjoy what you're doing; you have to be consumed by it. That's why I tell people to get involved with something they really believe in."

LIFE BEGINS AT RETIREMENT

Maggie Kuhn agrees that it's vitally important for older people to have a goal or purpose.

"Retirement can be a liberating force in your life; you're free from the restrictive structure of your job— free to take risks, to speak out, to do things that you couldn't do when you were responsible to a boss or a company," she says.

And like Jack LaLanne, Maggie isn't just talking: She was forced to retire in 1970 when she reached 65 years of age. At first she was depressed; she was taking care of her mother and brother at home and was scared that that was all she had left in life.

Then she met a woman who was taking care of her 99-year-old mother at home, "and she had the same anxiety." They talked about the limitations of being old. And they planned how to break out of them. As a first step, they formed a group of older people dedicated to battling injustice and joined the movement to end the war in Vietnam. They didn't just stuff envelopes or man the phone lines—they marched, they demonstrated, they got themselves arrested.

In 1970 Maggie Kuhn was told she was too old to keep her job; in 1971 she founded the Gray Panthers organization. Since then she's written books, lectured, organized and received a slew of prestigious awards. By 1978, the World Almanac had named her one of the "25 most influential women in America." She was soon to turn 80 when we spoke with her; it was a conversation vibrant and full of energy. "It's kind of a dull week if I don't have a good new idea," she says.

And she had plenty of good ideas about keeping your energy forever.

"First," she explained, "I don't tell people to 'stay young'—I tell them to stay alive, energized, hopeful and directed. Human energy has to be refueled. It's essential to have a purpose that's beyond your own self-interest. Public interest is ultimately more satisfying than self-interest."

She explains that one of the deepest pits in "the senior trap" is the loneliness and isolation many older people fall into. "I'm very opposed to senior communities," she explains, feeling that they offer no life, no stimulation.

Her energy, she feels, comes from "a continuous association with people of *all* ages, particularly young people," and she has some advice on how others can get started along the same road.

"If an older person's friendship circle was composed only of people from work or in the family, they're going to end up alone—and then they start to develop physical ailments from lack of human communication. There has to be a conscious reaching out to people of different ages, different points of view," she says.

Her advice? Get involved. "Go to the nearest college or university and enroll in a course," she suggests.

"Even if you've been ill and had problems dealing with doctors and hospitals, you can become a patient advocate and try to help others—or maybe even turn the system around. If you're on a fixed income and frightened to death about rising prices, become a watchdog over a public utility—make a fulltime vocation of watching them.

"Don't agonize," she says firmly, "*organize*! Turn your weaknesses, your needs, into strength and energy. Not only will it change you for the better, it'll change the things around you."

George Bernard Shaw once said that "men do not live long enough. They are, for all purposes of higher civilization, mere children when they die."

National Energy

One person can achieve almost anything once they set their mind—and energy—to a goal. Just imagine the accomplishments that are possible when an entire nation of people pools its energy resources and sets its sights on a dream. Suddenly, what had previously seemed an impossible task becomes a shining symbol of human endeavor.

The Road to Brasilia

It had been a dream since the late 1700s: an inland capital in the center of Brazil. But it was the spring of 1956 before construction began on a bleak and barren plain 500 miles from nowhere that would become the site of the city of Brasilia.

Just to get to the site, it was necessary to build hundreds of miles of roads through areas that hadn't yet been mapped. The hardwood forests were difficult to fell and the constant danger from poisonous snakes made supplies of antivenin a strong priority. In the first 20 months, 12 million cubic feet of earth were excavated and better than 534 miles of road were built. Eventually, a mammoth 1,350-mile road was finished, linking Brasilia with Belem, a major port at the mouth of the Amazon. Still, there was no lake, so they built an artificial one, as well as a championship golf course, hospitals, a university, museums and government buildings.

Hundreds of thousands of natives faced great hardships and almost impossible journeys, selling everything they owned to move through the wilderness because they believed in Brasilia. Without *their* energy, it would have remained a barren plateau.

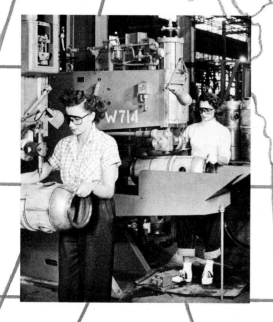

WW II: An Arsenal of Democracy

When America entered World War II with a vengeance following the destruction of Pearl Harbor, 135 million peaceful men and women were transformed into the most efficient fighting force the world has ever seen. Thirteen million entered the armed forces, 60 million took over the home front production lines, and enough poured their life savings into war bonds to bring in almost $200 billion. Forty-eight million joined the Red Cross and a blood donor drive became the biggest achievement in medical history, with 10 million American donations. Approximately 200,000 American industries "went to war," creating an army of workers greater than the number of soldiers fighting for all sides combined. Six million farms also joined the battle, and organized labor made the ultimate sacrifice by giving up their right to strike for the duration. The net results broke all world production records—and won the war.

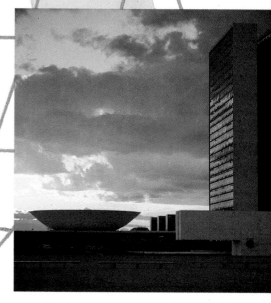

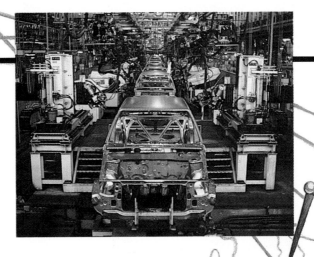

Egypt's Big Moving Day

The Egyptian king Ramses II has been called Ramses the Great, largely due to the phenomenal amount of temple building that took place during his reign. One of the most impressive projects was the construction of 2 temples at Abu Simbel on the Nile in 1250 B.C. Four colossal statues of Ramses guard the entrance to the main temple, which itself was carved out of sandstone cliff on the river's west bank.

In the 1960s, over a million unusable acres were reclaimed as a result of the Aswan High Dam project and it seemed certain that the temples were fated to wind up at the bottom of the reservoir created by the dam. But the Egyptian government and the United Nations Educational, Scientific and Cultural Organization sponsored a project that saved the temples. In what has been called the most dramatic rescue operation of its time, an international team of workers, engineers and scientists spent 2 years digging away the top of the cliff, sawing the temples and their statues into giant blocks and then reassembling both structures some 200 feet higher up, where they would be safe from the waters. More than 50 countries raised the funds for the project, making this mammoth effort of preservation an example of truly *inter*national energy.

Japan—One People, One Goal

Less than 25 years after their crushing defeat in World War II, Japan had risen to become the world's third leading economic power. It boasted the fastest (bullet) trains, the largest (9 million copies a day) newspaper, the biggest cargo ships and blast furnaces and the most expensive real estate in the world. This nation, which has literally rebuilt itself by demolishing entire mountains and using them to add land mass where once there was only sea, now leads the world in the production of sophisticated electronic equipment. All this in a land with practically no natural resources to speak of! A nation that already possessed a legendary zeal for work became dedicated to what foreign correspondent Robert Guillain called "the golden rule of the new Japan: all for the economy." So dedicated were these workers rushing to make their nation Number 1 by the year 2,000 that it was late in the 1960s before they borrowed a word from the French to fill a gap in their own language—"vacation."

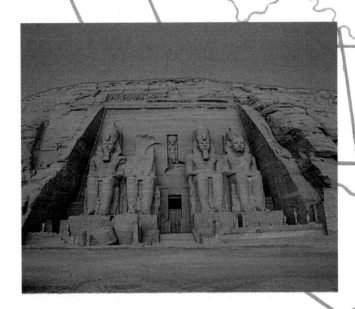

What's Your Energy Quotient?

You know what energy is and where it comes from in the body. You've seen examples of energetic people, energetic nations, and the amazing things you can accomplish with the right energy behind you. The question is—just how much energy is behind *you*? No, don't turn around! Face front and take this remarkably unscientific quiz to find your place in the wonderful world of energy.

1 It's 3:00 on an average weekday afternoon. How do you feel?
a. in good spirits
b. a little groggy
c. not sure because you're sound asleep

2 It's time to get out of bed in the morning. You:
a. can't wait to face the day
b. can take or leave the day
c. would like to pay someone to get out of bed and face the day for you

3 It's Sunday afternoon. You're going to:
a. indulge in some sort of fitness activity or work around the house
b. attend a sporting event or go somewhere with the family
c. become one with the living room couch

4 How do you feel about exercising for a half hour at least three times a week?
a. you already exercise that much
b. the idea is certainly not comfortable, but you think you can do it
c. it's something to be avoided at all costs

5 You're in a large department store. There's an escalator right next to a flight of stairs. You:
a. take the stairs
b. thank scientific progress for the escalator
c. decide to just shop on the first floor

6 On the average week night, which sounds most like you?
a. you get a "second wind" and get involved in something, be it mental, physical or social
b. you wind down to a good movie on TV starting at about 9:00 P.M.
c. you wind down to whatever happens to be on the TV starting at about 5:30 P.M.

7 Which sounds the most like you on a weekend night?
a. you go to a big party with lots of dancing
b. you'd prefer a small party with little or no dancing
c. you wind down to whatever happens to be on the TV starting at around noon

8 Speaking of television, just how much do you watch every day?
a. 2 hours or less
b. 3 hours or less
c. glued to the tube

9 When you watch TV, you:
a. are always jumping up to do things or are working on something else simultaneously
b. are sometimes distracted, but watch a few choice shows intently
c. don't want to miss one action-packed minute (if it wasn't for the bathroom run during commercials you'd probably explode)

10 When it comes to playing games or outdoor activities, you consider yourself:
a. an amateur athlete
b. a weekend warrior
c. a serious spectator

11 When your extended family gets together for reunions or holidays, the atmosphere is:
a. highly charged with lots of physical activity
b. filled with animated conversation
c. if you look real carefully, you can actually see people moving

12 How would you describe your parents and/or grandparents?
a. on the go all the time
b. achieved what they set out to in life
c. were content to take what came their way

13

Just in terms of energy levels, which kind of personality would you most identify with?
a. a hard-charging professional athlete
b. an actor or singer on Broadway
c. a lounge act that puts the room to sleep by 11:00 P.M.

14

You visit an ocean-front resort on vacation. You spend much of your time:
a. swimming, boating and enjoying the water (or walking on the beach)
b. reading on the beach while soaking up the rays in preparation for a big night on the town
c. sleeping on the beach all day in preparation for a night in the hotel bar

15

You've been putting together a presentation for work for months. The day before it's due, you're told to forget it. You:
a. either make the presentation to a select group anyway or use the ideas somewhere else
b. simply accept the situation and move on to the next job
c. are tremendously relieved because you weren't anywhere near ready yet

16

To you, retirement is:
a. a time of unlimited options
b. just another stage of life
c. slow death

17

You're absolutely pooped. It's entirely up to you whether you stop what you're doing or continue. You:
a. get away from what you're doing and go for a short walk, do some stretching or calisthenics or just get some fresh air before returning
b. stop what you're working on and switch to doing something different for awhile
c. stop what you're doing and curl up for a nice long nap

18

How's your sex life?
a. frequent and fun
b. totally predictable
c. negligible and narcoleptic

19

What's your idea of a nice long walk?
a. an all-day stroll
b. a morning or afternoon jaunt
c. getting up to change channels on the TV

20

When someone tries to get you to do something that you've never done before, you:
a. can't wait to savor this new experience
b. are a little anxious, but ready to try
c. have to wash your hair

21

How well do you sleep?
a. soundly and always wake up refreshed
b. sometimes restless, but mostly pretty well
c. you fight to the death with tangled, sweaty sheets every night

22

How would you rate your recovery time after an illness or accident?
a. excellent—right back on your feet
b. average—give yourself time to recover
c. poor—malingering is considered an art

23

How often do you laugh?
a. always laughing and smiling
b. like to hear a good joke—or tell one
c. bah, humbug

24

How about if the joke's on *you*?
a. if it's funny—laugh
b. grin and bear it
c. harbor sinister designs toward the jokester

25

How do you react to mental challenge—say a difficult but rewarding book or game of chess?
a. thrive on such challenges
b. try to do your best
c. have to wash your hair

26

American author William James said that "it is only by risking our persons from one hour to another that we live at all." How do you feel about that?
a. you agree—a life without risks is really no life at all
b. it's good to feel that way occasionally, but you prefer to pick and choose your risks
c. what was he, nuts?

2

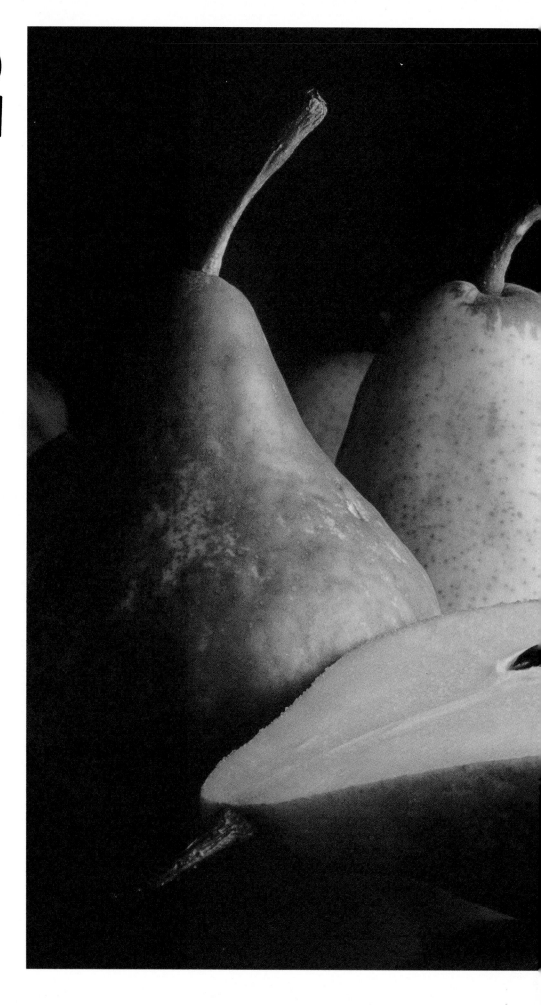

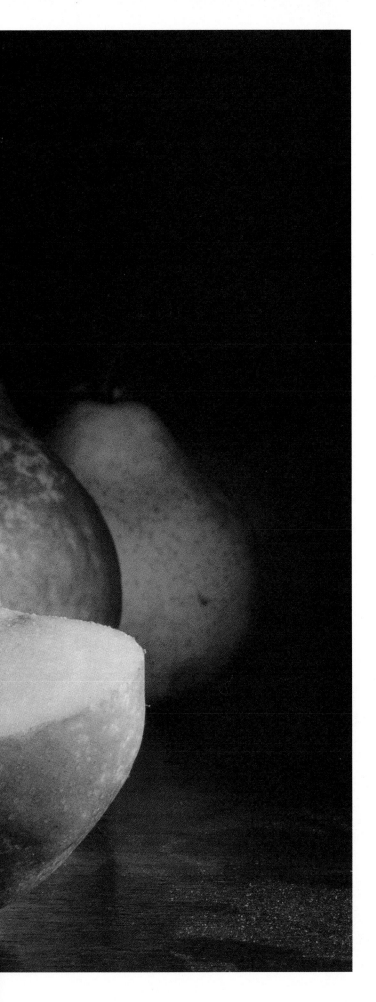

Food: Fuel for the Busy Body

You can say yes, yes to some former no-nos, as long as you follow this advice: If it makes you feel good, it's probably good for you.

Historians say that three major scientific discoveries have seriously shaken mankind's cherished assumptions: Copernicus's disclosure that the earth wasn't the center of the universe; Darwin's telling us the apes were our ancestors; and Freud's unveiling of the subconscious as a major factor in our behavior.

Nutrition experts may very well add a fourth discovery to this list—that starches (complex carbohydrates) like potatoes don't *always* provide steady energy and that sugars (simple carbohydrates) like those in a candy bar don't *always* give a quick lift, followed by an equally quick drop.

"For many years it had been assumed that carbohydrates behave in predictable ways," says Phyllis A. Crapo, a registered dietitian and an assistant adjunct professor of nutrition at the University of California. Complex carbohydrates were believed to be slowly digested and absorbed, causing a gradual rise in glucose levels, the body's chief source of energy. On the other hand, simple carbohydrates [such as sugar and fruit] were assumed to be readily digested and absorbed, producing large and rapid increases in glucose levels.

What did this mean in terms of the scientific understanding of your energy levels? Simple carbohydrates were thought to be a little like the drug "speed," causing quick, crazy ups and devastating downs. The energy from complex carbohydrates was thought to be like a happy marriage—steady, constant, smooth.

Solid theory. It told us that candy bars and doughnuts were energy no-nos and that brown rice and beans were as suited to our bodies as an old flannel shirt. But theory isn't always fact. How

Grazing: Energy to Go

What do the slender beauties of Bali and today's active people have in common? They always seem to be eating—but only a handful at a time.

Grazing, as it's called, is sort of a throwback to our primitive urge to scavenge, say anthropologists. You nibble as you go, but consciously choose foods with nutrient quality.

One step beyond fast foods, these light, ready-to-eat snacks consist of such things as nachos, potato skins, fresh fruit cups, "gourmet" popcorn and raw vegetables and dips.

There's some evidence that several small meals eaten throughout the day are handled better by the body than three big meals. Nibbling nutritiously keeps blood sugar levels on an even keel, helping to avoid energy deficits.

many of us have eaten a doughnut and felt *better*—or at least not worse? Or eaten a dinner with beans and rice as the main course and felt sleepy and too full. Common sense tells us that our response to food is individual. We aren't test tubes—there are no standard reactions to the (food) chemicals put into us. We're people, each with a unique set of genes and food preferences, and our diet for top-level energy should be just that: personal, unique, ours. And that's what the new studies on carbohydrates are telling us.

A study conducted by Ms. Crapo and her colleagues, for example, showed that potato starch turned into glucose almost as quickly as pure sugar. In a second study, David J. A. Jenkins of the University of Toronto and Thomas M. S. Wolever of Oxford showed that a bowl of ice cream or a sampling of fructose (the type of sugar found in fruit) may increase blood sugar only a little, while carrots, a slice of bread or a potato can send it soaring. It depends on a lot of factors, including *who* is eating the food.

A third study not only retired the old beliefs about carbohydrates—it buried them. John P. Bantle, M.D., and his colleagues at the University of Minnesota showed that even replacing all the wheat in a meal with table sugar made little difference in glucose levels.

What these studies reveal, says Ms. Crapo, is that the body's responses to food are far more complex and individual than had been previously appreciated.

YUPPIES' YUMMIES

An article in the *New York Times* that detailed the diets of successful young professionals showed just how diverse—yet effective—eating styles can be. A 29-year-old vice president of Sotheby's—the world's most prestigious auction house, selling million-dollar items almost daily—starts his day with a high-protein drink that he describes as "a sort of grown-up baby formula."

A professional "bodyworker," specializing in massage therapies like shiatsu, eats a late breakfast of Chinese take-out food. And skips lunch.

An investment banker also skips lunch. And breakfast. But he does well on "nibbles of this and that" throughout his 12-hour day.

A self-described entrepreneur lives on three or four frozen food entrees a day.

This doesn't mean that what many still think of as "healthy eating" is passé. Whole foods like lean meats, grains, fruits, vegetables and low-fat dairy products are the type of fuel the body seems to crave. The lesson here is that no *one* food is "bad" or "good." It's your *total* diet—customized according to your preferences and personality—that makes the difference.

HOW DANCERS STAY ON THEIR TOES

That's also the viewpoint of Lilian Cheung, D.Sc., a registered dietitian and executive director of Medical Nutrition Associates in Boston. Dr. Cheung is emphatic that there are only individual eating styles for high energy, not universal rules. Her nutritional philosophy has its proving ground with some of the most energy-demanding bodies around—the members of the Boston Ballet School, to whom she is nutritional adviser.

Dr. Cheung tailors her nutritional counseling to the energy needs of the dancers. "I recommend certain things before a performance—they can't have a full stomach, they can't have a big meal 1 to 2 hours before they dance."

Although Dr. Cheung recognizes that her dancers must eat according to personal lifestyle and daily demands ("most of them are snackers rather than meal eaters," she says), she applies some general guidelines, too. "A diet low in fat, high in complex carbohydrates, with lots of vegetables and fruits and a good amount of protein is a very healthy diet," she says.

Dr. Cheung's own life is quite demanding, but her diet and eating patterns help keep energy levels high. "I eat three meals a day—not big ones—and I snack in between. I

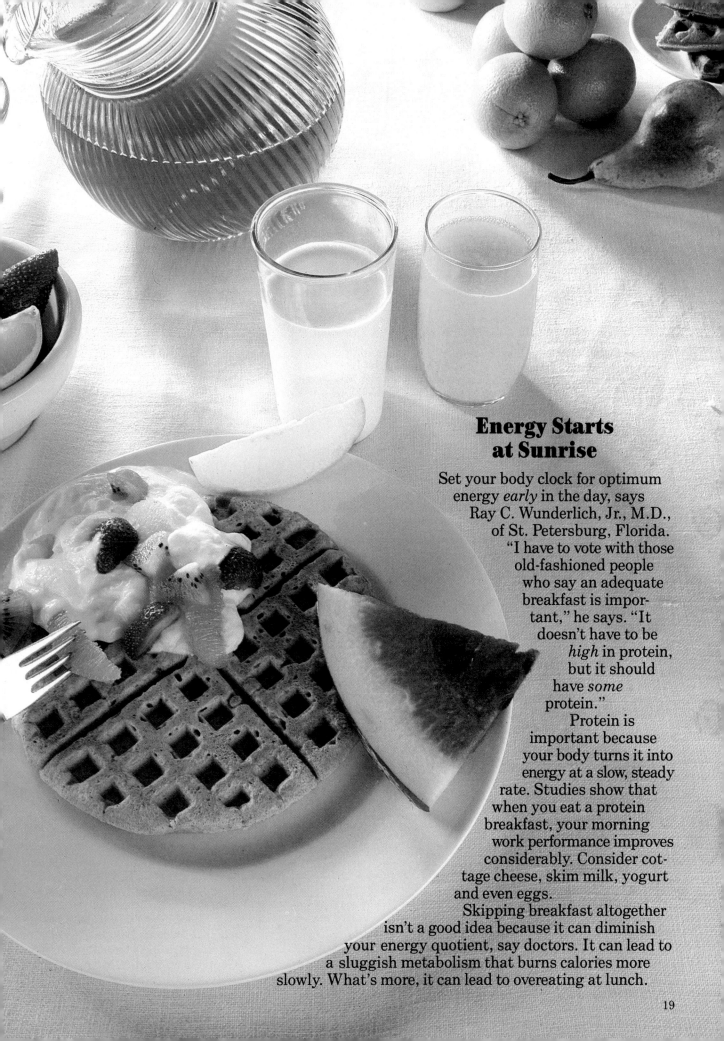

Energy Starts at Sunrise

Set your body clock for optimum energy *early* in the day, says Ray C. Wunderlich, Jr., M.D., of St. Petersburg, Florida. "I have to vote with those old-fashioned people who say an adequate breakfast is important," he says. "It doesn't have to be *high* in protein, but it should have *some* protein."

Protein is important because your body turns it into energy at a slow, steady rate. Studies show that when you eat a protein breakfast, your morning work performance improves considerably. Consider cottage cheese, skim milk, yogurt and even eggs.

Skipping breakfast altogether isn't a good idea because it can diminish your energy quotient, say doctors. It can lead to a sluggish metabolism that burns calories more slowly. What's more, it can lead to overeating at lunch.

19

don't believe what most diet books say about snacks. They're fine as long as they're healthful. I am not a big dessert eater, but when I see something attractive like a fruit tart with kiwi, I will eat it. But I won't eat it every day."

But food isn't the only factor in the diet/energy equation. What you *think* about your food also affects how energetic—or tired—it makes you feel.

"The way food makes you feel has a lot to do with your expectations—what you've been conditioned to believe will happen when you eat it," says Dr. Bantle.

"In large measure, your expectations determine your reaction to foods," agrees John Hennessy, Ph.D., a psychologist from New Jersey.

If you think that potatoes are a *bad* food, for example (a perception many dieters have), then your response to eating potatoes will probably be low energy. It's a sort of self-fulfilling prophecy.

So how can you be a prophet of high energy?

"Any *extreme* feelings about eating will ultimately be energy sapping," says Dr. Hennessy. He counsels a kind of dietary self-love—that we should see *all* food as a way to nourish and support ourselves, not withhold food as a punishment or eat it guiltily as if it were a sin. "Use food as a daily opportunity to feel good." And that means any food, including one that's almost impossible to avoid—sugar.

HIGH-OCTANE FUEL

A bold statement? Not at all. After all, how many times have you met someone who claims to hate sugar? Probably never. We feel pretty safe in saying that just about everybody enjoys sweet treats. Their reputation as "forbidden foods" only makes them all the more alluring. In fact, our desire for a quick surge of energy is often our best excuse to eat them. Take this scenario as an example:

It's 10:30 A.M. You've been slaving over your report. Suddenly your concentration wanes and your thoughts turn to the snack machines in the company lunchroom. You're grumpy and frazzled. You *know* a sugary Danish will improve your mood *and* give you the mental energy to complete your report by lunchtime. You go for it.

This midmorning letdown is all too familiar to many of us—an unwelcome interruption in the smooth flow of the workday. Efficiency and production *should* be cresting at midmorning, then gradually declining toward noon. But instead, many of us plummet into the blahs. What's responsible for this phenomenon, and—more important—how can we avoid it?

It is caused by a drop in blood sugar levels and bad episodes can be prevented simply by eating wisely, says David Shearer, M.D., endocrinologist at York Hospital in York,

---

How to Beat the 3 O'Clock Blahs

Scientists call it the postprandial (after eating) dip. Eating the wrong foods at the wrong time is part of the cause and a marked ebb in energy and work efficiency is the unwanted effect.

If afternoon fatigue has traditionally been a problem for you, one obvious solution is to eat light at lunch. Digestion requires energy, so by loading yourself down with a full-course meal at noon, you're giving yourself "extra" work that takes energy away from your job.

Besides avoiding a mammoth lunch, try not to make a habit of going to bed too late. The most important hours for sleep are between 10:00 P.M. and midnight, says Ray C. Wunderlich, M.D., of St. Petersburg, Florida. If your body operates on the typical day-person's cycle, these are the hours of sleep that pay off during the afternoon of the next day.

Some business executives have tailored their own solutions to avoid the afternoon dip. One Fortune 500 company founder says if he feels drowsiness coming on he simply stands up—especially if it's in a dull meeting.

A famous Texas oilman says he's never experienced a 3 o'clock slump, because his business is much too exciting. Love of job, he says, creates its own energy. Perhaps his is the best antidote of all.

Pennsylvania. The right breakfast, for example, can prevent the slumps, technically known as rebound hypoglycemia.

SUGAR AS "BRAIN FOOD"

"This effect is a perfectly normal reaction," says Dr. Shearer. "Your body is very well tuned to keeping your blood sugar [glucose] at certain levels. The reason for this is that your brain runs on sugar—it won't run on any other fuel. The body is organized to maintain a flow of glucose to your brain. It will take glucose from food or from body stores in the liver or muscle and put it into your bloodstream and send it to your brain."

Here's how the process works. "After you eat, the level of sugar in the blood goes up, then the insulin level also goes up, allowing the blood sugar to be absorbed and utilized," Dr. Shearer says. "That taken care of, the blood sugar level goes down." This process sometimes causes side effects—you know, nervousness, jumpiness, the frazzles.

"When people talk about having this kind of reaction," says Dr. Shearer, "what they're experiencing is a reaction to having too much sugar on an empty stomach. You take that same amount of sugar and put it at the end of a meal, say as dessert, and you won't have that reaction because the stomach is filled with a lot of different foods that take a long time to be broken down and absorbed."

What exactly does all this mean to the executive who has just pumped two quarters into the vending machine? It means he or she is on a carousel ride of ups and downs. Coffee and a doughnut for breakfast can perk you up at 8:00 A.M. and bottom you out at 10:30. A new infusion of sugar—a Danish, for example—can take you through the same cycle during late morning. "The absorption of sugar is dependent on how much is in the stomach at the time you eat that Danish or candy bar or whatever it is," Dr. Shearer reiterates.

The obvious answer, then, is to eat a better breakfast. "I usually recommend eating a balanced diet, not stressing any one group of foods

Sustenance for Success

Time magazine described him as "one of the most famous and controversial businessmen in the U.S. . . . who has reaped his vast payoffs through the mastery of the takeover battle." He's T. Boone Pickens, chairman of Mesa Petroleum in Amarillo, Texas, a maverick business tycoon with a voice like warmed honey and the reputation of "a sneaky poker player, a veritable rattlesnake in the woodpile."

His ruthless shake-ups of corporate America are just the kind of wily behavior you'd expect from someone bred on the macho chow of Texas prime beef. But wait a second. The man who is nimbly rearranging the map of corporate America makes no such claims. In fact, by his own admission, his diet is generally as modest as his takeovers are grandiose.

Does orange juice, a few cups of hot lemon water and a bowl of cereal sound like the breakfast of a champion? Well, it is. "Sometimes I like some real toasty whole wheat bread with melted Swiss cheese," confesses the corporate raider.

Lunch, which is often served in flight aboard his private jet, may be a broiled, lean hamburger—no bread—fruit and sometimes frozen yogurt for dessert. Dinner is often soup and salad, says the man who also runs, plays racquetball and sleeps only 5 to 6 hours a night.

"I'm not a health nut," says the mild-mannered Texan, "but I've always believed everything should be in moderation." (Except mergers.)

If you have any doubt that most high-powered executives operate on similar fare, listen to what another says.

Bob Garten, vice president of Catalytica Associates, a fast-growing technology development company in Palo Alto, California, starts his day at 6:00 A.M. After an hour of race-walking he sits down to a breakfast of mixed whole grain cereals with "a couple tablespoons of raw bran, a dash of wheat germ, a dash of brewer's yeast" and low-fat milk. "I usually eat half of a banana, strawberries or raspberries," he says. Lunch is yogurt or turkey, lettuce and tomato on whole wheat, followed by carrot and celery sticks.

For a business luncheon, "I avoid steaks and pork chops and order plain broiled fish. I sometimes splurge and ask for a little sauce. Generally I don't drink liquor, because it makes me drowsy," says Garten.

over any other. And mix them up," Dr. Shearer says.

Will someone who claims to have not just a sweet tooth but sweet *teeth* have to give up brownies, sweet rolls and crullers? Not necessarily, says the doctor. "For people who like to eat sweets, in general I recommend that you take them in moderation on a *full* stomach. That way you won't get the big rebound."

USE, DON'T ABUSE

A lot of people never experience such a crash into total fatigue. Nevertheless, they are still looking to improve their level of energy.

Bill, for example, works hard in his office all day, yet he's really pretty sedentary—until lunch hour, that is, when he burns up the court, competing with other top-level players at racquetball.

And then there's Carol, mother of two little boys who are always on the go. In addition to chasing after them she puts in the usual round of cooking, laundry, dusting, vacuuming, gardening, mowing, painting and fixing up. She usually doesn't sit down until after the boys' bedtime, when she drops exhausted onto the sofa.

Bill demands his energy in short spurts while Carol needs lesser amounts sustained all day long.

Both of these people can meet their energy needs by manipulating the types of carbohydrates in their diets. To do so successfully, they'll first need to know something about the nature of carbohydrates and how they convert to the sugar, or glucose, that the body uses for energy. Table sugar and the types of sugar found in fruit, milk and pastries, and to some degree in vegetables, are simple carbohydrates. They're called simple because—molecularly speaking— that's exactly what they are. There are not many chemical bonds to be broken before a simple carbohydrate

is absorbed by the bloodstream, so it is converted quickly.

Complex carbohydrates, such as those found in potatoes and pasta, are made up of hundreds of molecules linked together. They take longer to digest and thus take longer for your body to break down into a usable form of sugar.

If you are like Bill the racquetball player, you may benefit from getting a quick kick of energy from a food containing a simple carbohydrate. A handful of raisins or dates—or, let's face it, even a candy bar—can give him the power to play hard through a lunch-hour game. Carol, on the other hand, would probably benefit from getting her energy by eating the complex carbohydrate foods. Despite the new findings of the nutritional *avant garde*, most doctors still recommend this division of labor for simple and complex carbohydrates.

"There are foods with quick energy versus those that supply intermediate or long-term energy," says Allen McDaniels, M.D., of San Pedro, California. "An athlete who requires a burst of energy requires more simple sugars, which burn quickly without turning to fat. Simple sugars are used when you want energy *right now*. Suppose you're hiking, for example. You'll want to carry a chocolate bar or an orange or something that has a pretty high percentage of simple sugars.

"On the other hand, someone doing office work, for example, requires complex carbohydrates and protein so they can have *sustained* energy rather than needing readily available high bursts of energy," he explains.

As for snacks, Dr. McDaniels recommends fruits. "If I'm doing heavy physical exercise I like to have a light midmorning snack and a light afternoon snack as well. I prefer eating fruits that grow in the temperate climate—apples, pears, berries— and stay away from tropical fruits like bananas, which are high in sugar. I'd also go easy on raisins or dates because they too are high in sugars and unless you're going to expend a lot of energy, they'll be stored as fat."

THE COMPLEX MADE SIMPLE

In addition to the sugars found in foods, there are also the sugars we add to foods. Table sugar, for example, has a very bad reputation, even though it is no better or worse than many other sweeteners, while others have undeservedly good reputations. Here's the rundown of what's available.

Sucrose. This is the chemical name for table sugar, which is made by putting sugar beets or sugar cane through a rigorous refinement procedure. Chemically, it is made up of equal parts of glucose and fructose.

Fructose. It is identical to table sugar in calorie content, but it is 70 percent sweeter. It is thought to be less attractive to tooth-decay bacteria than regular sugar.

Brown sugar. White sugar with a tan.

Honey. A hodgepodge of sugars. Its precise makeup of fructose, glucose, maltose and sucrose depends on the combination of nectars the bees have used.

Molasses. This is a component of sugar beets and sugar cane that's removed in the refining process. It is rich in minerals, among them chromium, iron, calcium, potassium and magnesium. It has more calories than sugar and portion for portion is not as sweet.

Yet sugar isn't the only thing people gravitate to when they are looking for that kick to make it through the day. The other—and perhaps even more popular—standby is coffee.

Yes! Candy Can Give You Energy

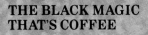

It's 30 minutes before the big game and the athlete gobbles a candy bar, hoping for an extra burst of energy from the sugar. He should have waited until half-time.

Ellen Coleman, a Riverside, California, dietitian and exercise physiologist, says that sugar eaten *before* exercise can actually impair energy by causing a large release of insulin, a hormone that limits your body's ability to use its fat stores for energy. But, she explains, eating a candy bar *during* activity is another story. "Exercise suppresses insulin release," she says, so that nothing cancels out the sugar, which converts quickly into fuel for pep.

THE BLACK MAGIC THAT'S COFFEE

Some people like to start the day with it. Others can't end a meal without it. Its aroma can compete with the world's best perfumes. It has no calories, yet its flavor is rich. All in all, coffee is hard to beat as a wonderful refreshment.

Yet, many people who love— really *love*—coffee, limit themselves to a cup a day. They do so because they know their limit. And that, in a nutshell, is the secret to healthful coffee drinking.

Healthful? Coffee? Although in recent years some scientists have considered the brew to be simmering with potential health hazards, coffee is enjoying some revisionist thinking

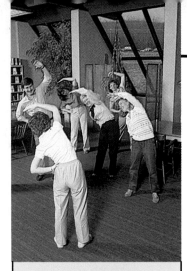

Let's Take a Noncoffee Break

First get together your noncoffee survival kit: a comfortable pair of walking shoes, a tape player with earphones, or a snack. Push your coffee cup aside at break time and grab any one of the above.

What more need be said for the invigorating effects of the fresh dose of oxygen you'll get from a brisk walk, or the extra pep you'll feel after a few minutes of stretching? Not in the mood for exercise? Then find a quiet spot, don your earphones and turn on the music you know will stimulate yet relax you. Or try a high-energy snack, such as cheese, peanut butter crackers or a piece of fruit.

these days. It may not be as bad as you once thought—provided, of course, you practice moderation. In fact, you might be the best judge of how "good" coffee is for you and how much is too much.

The source of controversy over coffee is its most studied (though not necessarily largest) constituent, caffeine. Generally considered to be the most widely used drug in America and Europe, caffeine is an often powerful central nervous system stimulant that, in some people, can cause modest increases in blood pressure and heart rate, arrhythmias, anxiety and sleeplessness.

For most people, caffeine taken in modest amounts is a pretty harmless and pleasurable vice. "If you're a normal person, your body can cope with 300 milligrams of caffeine a day—that's about three cups of coffee," says Manfred Kroger, Ph.D., professor of food science at Pennsylvania State University and a spokesman for the Institute of Food Technologists.

He cautions, however, that coffee, which contains literally hundreds of less-studied chemicals in addition to caffeine, can be ambrosia to one person and hemlock to another. Response can be as individual as fingerprints.

"I, for instance, am not a 'normal' person," says Dr. Kroger. "If I drink three cups of coffee in the afternoon, I'll be up until midnight. If I drink one cup after six, I'll be up until three. I haven't given up coffee entirely. I've learned to work around my sensitivity."

Most people do. Coffee has a way of tipping off the body when enough is enough. "It seems that if you take too much you tend not to take any more," says Peter Dews, M.D., Ph.D., professor of psychiatry and psychobiology at Harvard Medical School and editor of *Caffeine, Perspectives from Recent Research.* "Suppose, for instance, you drink coffee during a business meeting. If you start feeling uncomfortable, you stop. That's why you see so many half-drunk cups of coffee lying around after meetings in a way you rarely see half-drunk cups of soft drinks. At a subliminal level, there's an automatic stop with coffee. You don't even have to think about it."

WHEN ENOUGH IS ENOUGH

But a lot of people *are* thinking about it. And one of their greatest concerns has to do with side effects.

The most common side effects of coffee are nervousness and insomnia, and whether you experience them depends largely on how much caffeine you're getting and your individual susceptibility. You'll have to let your past coffee experiences be your guide.

"Your body will tell you," says Dr. Kroger. "People should learn to observe their bodies the way they do their cars."

Your body, like your car, can have its knocks and pings. You may be drinking too much coffee if you're unusually nervous, restless or battling with insomnia—that's the old coffee jitters. You could also be overdosing if you're experiencing heart palpitations, diarrhea, headache or heartburn. In some people, coffee acts as a diuretic, so you may have increased urine output.

Quantitatively, excessive consumption can be considered anything over ten cups of strongly brewed coffee a day, which can lead to what doctors call caffeinism. The symptoms are identical to—and sometimes mistaken for—anxiety neurosis. Caffeinism affects as many as one in ten people.

How caffeine affects you personally may depend on your own metabolism or whether you drink coffee on a regular basis. One of the problems researchers face when studying the effects of caffeine on humans is that it affects habitual consumers and nonconsumers quite differently, say caffeine researchers Peter Curatolo, M.D., and David Robertson, M.D.

For instance, when a group of people who did not drink coffee was given a daily dose of 250 milligrams of caffeine (equivalent to about 2½ cups of coffee), these so-called caffeine-naive people experienced small increases in blood pressure, heart rate and excretions of stress hormones from the adrenal gland. So did a group of habitual drinkers—who had abstained for three weeks before the test—when they were given 250 milligrams of caffeine three times a day for a week. The difference, however, was that the habitual drinkers developed a tolerance to the caffeine long before the week was up and no longer had any untoward reactions.

THE COFFEE QUESTIONNAIRE

Here are some of the most common questions coffee drinkers ask.

Will Coffee Keep Me Up at Night?
Your metabolism—specifically, how quickly your system eliminates caffeine—may determine whether coffee keeps you up at night. In a study at Jerusalem's Hadassah University Hospital, researchers found that people who said coffee kept them up consumed less coffee—because of their bad reaction to it—and eliminated it more slowly from their systems than people who claimed coffee didn't affect their sleep.

The researchers concluded that individual metabolism dictates whether coffee will rob you of a good night's sleep or not bother you at all.

Why Do I Drink Coffee? It may be because of the taste or because of the nice buzz it gives you, making you feel that "God's in his heaven and all's right with the world."

In a Swiss study, volunteers who drank the equivalent of one cup of coffee said they felt full of ideas, vigor, alertness and energy. Other researchers have found that caffeine can increase reading speed without increasing errors, improve the capacity for sustained intellectual effort and lead to less aggressive behaviors. There is even some indication that coffee increases aerobic capacity, which can give an athlete more staying power.

But be forewarned: What coffee giveth, coffee may take away. Some people experience a poststimulation letdown that can make them as tired and lethargic as they were alert and energetic. One problem you can face if you treat coffee as more than simply a satisfying beverage is that you'll start to reach for more than

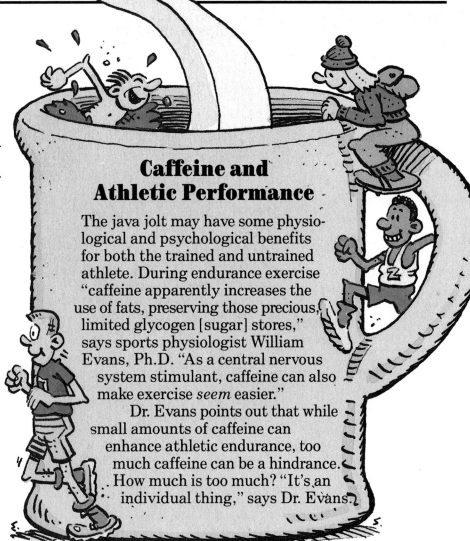

Caffeine and Athletic Performance

The java jolt may have some physiological and psychological benefits for both the trained and untrained athlete. During endurance exercise "caffeine apparently increases the use of fats, preserving those precious, limited glycogen [sugar] stores," says sports physiologist William Evans, Ph.D. "As a central nervous system stimulant, caffeine can also make exercise *seem* easier."

Dr. Evans points out that while small amounts of caffeine can enhance athletic endurance, too much caffeine can be a hindrance. How much is too much? "It's an individual thing," says Dr. Evans.

you can handle just to prolong the kick.

Are There Any Long-Term Health Effects from Drinking Coffee? Early studies linked caffeine with heart disease and cancer, but since then most of those findings have been disputed and most medical experts believe there's no clear evidence supporting them. But moderation is the key. A recent trial study on coffee's role in elevated cholesterol—considered to be a factor in heart disease—done at Stanford University, found that sedentary men between 30 and 55 who drink three cups of coffee a day might have a higher risk of developing heart disease than those who drink less coffee.

There is some indication that heavy coffee consumption, when accompanied by other diet and lifestyle

Going Light on Alcohol

Sometimes a drink or two is nice, but the tired-out feeling afterward is not. So when offered a choice of beer, wine or whiskey, you immediately think, "Aha, I'll take a beer and keep from getting drowsy." Well, consider the following and think again.

Beer contains 17.6 grams of pure alcohol to the 12-ounce bottle; a jigger of whiskey, 15 grams; and a glass of table wine, 9.9 grams.

Surprised? Even a "lite" beer has 3 more grams of alcohol than wine.

factors, may increase cholesterol levels, a finding of several previous studies done outside the United States. There was no such association found when the men in the Stanford study limited their coffee to two or fewer cups a day.

How Does Coffee Affect My Nutrition? There's some evidence that coffee can inhibit the absorption of both iron and thiamine (vitamin B_1). In the case of thiamine, it doesn't appear to be caffeine that's the culprit but another coffee chemical, chlorgenic acid, which can have an effect even if you drink decaffeinated coffee, because it is not eliminated during the decaffeinating process.

How Can I Enjoy Coffee without Worrying? Although moderation is the key to coffee comfort, for some the most logical step is to switch to decaffeinated coffee. Many people can't tell the difference between decaffeinated and the real thing. But if you can, you might want to stick to either instant or percolated coffee which, depending on how strong you make it, can contain less caffeine on average than drip coffee.

Adding milk to coffee won't cut down on caffeine, although it tends to slow its absorption. But cafe au lait, that delicious French way of serving coffee by filling half the cup with hot milk and half with dark coffee, will reduce the caffeine by reducing the amount of coffee in your cup. Substitute skim or low-fat milk and you eliminate calories and cholesterol as well.

LET'S HAVE A DRINK

Of course, the buzz you get from a cup of coffee isn't the kind you're looking for *after* work, when the goal is to unwind the body and drain the mind of the stresses of the day. Some people like to do it by reaching for a drink. And the invitation isn't only heard just after work. You hear it at ballgames, parties, dances, friends' homes—well, just about everywhere. "Let's have a drink" is a perfectly sociable and acceptable thing to do. But . . .

Is there a way to toast your friend's new job without feeling like a wrung-out dishcloth afterward? Can you split a bottle of wine with a client at lunch and not nod off at your desk later? Is it possible to savor the rich depth of cognac without conking out?

The answer is an emphatic *yes*. If you know how, you can drink without getting drunk and without losing your edge. In fact, drinking can work in your favor. It can loosen you up so that you are socially at ease and possibly even vivacious. Of course, the trick is knowing your limit. And to know that, you first need to know a little biology.

Have you ever noticed that one person can toss back three or four Scotch-and-waters and walk away clear of eye and steady of gait, while another poor soul will be babbling silliness after only one? Why the difference?

According to the National Institute on Alcohol Abuse and Alcoholism, the effects of alcohol depend not so much on how many drinks you have as on how fast the alcohol is absorbed into the blood and how quickly it can be eliminated from the body. In other words, it's quite one thing to drink three beers in the course of an entire evening and yet another to chug three beers in half an hour. The number of drinks is the same, but the level of alcohol in the blood would be significantly higher in the second case.

According to the institute, when people reach a blood alcohol concentration (BAC) of 0.10 percent—the legal limit for drunkenness in most states—voluntary motor actions usually become perceptibly clumsy. Also around this level the person takes slightly longer to react to a visual or auditory stimulus. You can be arrested for drunken driving if your drinking has caused the BAC to reach 0.10 percent. But higher concentrations are possible.

Again according to the institute, "At 0.20 percent the individual staggers and may lie down; he or she may be easily angered, shout or weep . . . At 0.30 percent the person commonly acts confused and may be stuporous." Stuporous, of course, is the opposite of energetic. It's pretty easy to see that if you can keep the concentration of alcohol in the blood on the low side, you can enjoy yourself without turning into a bar sponge.

WHAT'S YOUR BODY TYPE?

The first thing to take into account in safe drinking is your body size. The smaller you are, the more careful you have to be. The reason is again one of concentration, but this time not only in the blood. When alcohol finds its way into the bloodstream it eventually is distributed throughout the entire body—mixing with the water in all the tissues. Simply put, the bigger the body, the more water it contains and therefore the lower the concentration of alcohol. For large people, it's akin to pouring a shot of whiskey into an 8-ounce glass, while for small people it's like pouring that same size shot into a 6-ounce glass.

Women must be extra careful to monitor their drinking—not only because they are smaller than men but also because they have a friendly little layer of fat that men don't. The fat cells in that layer (or fat anywhere) contain very little water, thus forcing the alcohol to become even more concentrated in tissues that do hold water. The result can be the dreaded elevated blood alcohol concentration. In fact, the National Institute on Alcohol Abuse and Alcoholism says that if a man and woman of equal weight had the same number of drinks, the drinks would hit the woman harder.

Women also have additional concerns. They should be aware that in the time just before their menstrual period, their body burns up alcohol at a slower rate. And women taking oral contraceptives eliminate alcohol from the body at a lower rate. The wise woman who wants to drink should consider these three factors—size, cycle and contraceptive—when she enters the cocktail lounge.

THE DRINKER'S FORMULA

To keep yourself from dreading the day after the night before, be sure to follow these guidelines:

Know Your Limit

Body Weight (lb.)	Number of Drinks* during a 2-hour period									
100	1	2	3	4	5	6	7	8	9	10
120	1	2	3	4	5	6	7	8	9	10
140	1	2	3	4	5	6	7	8	9	10
160	1	2	3	4	5	6	7	8	9	10
180	1	2	3	4	5	6	7	8	9	10
200	1	2	3	4	5	6	7	8	9	10
220	1	2	3	4	5	6	7	8	9	10
240	1	2	3	4	5	6	7	8	9	10

Be Careful Driving BAC to .05%	Driving May Be Impaired .05-.09%	Do Not Drive .10% & Up

BAC—Blood Alcohol Content

*One drink is 1¼ oz. of 80-proof liquor, 12 oz. of beer or 4 oz. of wine

This chart provides averages only. Individuals may vary, and factors such as food in the stomach, medication and fatigue can affect your tolerance.

First of All, Dilute. If you lower the concentration of alcohol in your glass, it will enter your bloodstream more slowly. (A larger drink also takes longer to consume, a distinct benefit.) But when diluting, not just any mixer will do. A carbonated mixer—like seltzer or tonic—will speed alcohol into the blood. So will sparkling wine. On the other hand, sweet mixers slow absorption. Thus gin and orange juice, for example, might be a safer choice than gin and tonic, and Chablis could be a better choice than champagne.

The bigger they are the harder they fall? Not when it comes to liquor. The big bruiser's size is all in his favor when it comes to being able to hold his own in the cocktail lounge. All things being equal, over a 2-hour period the big guy can hold an average of 6 drinks to the 100-pound weakling's 2 drinks before they both pass into the twilight zone. But remember, this is only an average. Things like food consumption, fatigue, the proof of the alcohol and yes, even practice, are all controlling factors in keeping your pace and not getting drunk.

Be Sure to Eat. According to the institute, "eating just before or during drinking slows the absorption of alcohol, especially if the foods are high in oils or milk products." For safe drinking, be sure to ask your host to pass the cheese and crackers or the sour cream dip.

Pace Yourself. A normal, healthy man can thoroughly process a standard bar drink in about 2 hours. The alcohol is absorbed into the blood, circulated, then eliminated—some burned up for energy, some given off as carbon dioxide, and some used to form amino acids, carbohydrates and fats.

If one drink every 2 hours doesn't sound like a party pace, consider that this measure is for 1½ ounces of 80-proof whiskey. With enough cheese, crackers, mixers and ice you may be able to sneak in another drink—but only if you're willing to risk a case of the blahs.

OVEREATING, OVERWEIGHT

Of course the gin, orange juice, cheese, chips and dips all lead, almost inevitably, to one thing—fat. And even teetotalers are facing the same problem.

Furniture manufacturers say they are designing broader-bottomed chairs for our broader-bottomed citizens. Clothing manufacturers report that individuals of both sexes and all ages have shown an increase in body measurements.

It's awfully nice of these manufacturers to accommodate our widening girth, but how much healthier it would be if they had to make their products smaller instead. However, it's going to take a whale of a dose of will power to reverse America's overeating trend. According to the latest figures, 36 million Americans beyond age 20 are considered obese—that's 20 percent or more above normal weight. It's enough to put overeating up there as America's favorite pastime.

Yet, "if you look around and start identifying people who seem to be dynamos of energy," says Charles Kuntzleman, Ed.D., author of *Maximum Personal Energy*, "you would notice one thing: Most are slim and trim, with no protruding stomachs, no 'orange peel' skin, no flabby arms and spongy thighs. That in itself should tell you something about the relationship between energy and obesity."

There's no doubt about it. If you're carrying around a few extra pounds, you've got an "energy-robbing burden," says Dr. Kuntzleman. Would you tie a 5- or 10-pound cement block to your back and carry it around all day? If you did you'd realize how your muscles and bones labor under the strain of that extra weight. Your heart and lungs, too, must work harder to assist the muscles. Your blood pressure increases

---

High-Fat Foods

High fat means high calories. This list gives you an idea of some of the common foods that are high in fat. For effective weight loss, think twice—or better yet, half as much—about foods with more than 25 percent of their calories coming from fat.

Food	Percent of Calories from Fat
Oil	100.0
Butter	99.1
Mayonnaise	98.3
Margarine	98.2
Creamy dressing	88.8
Cream, light	87.9
Cream cheese	87.8
Sour cream	85.2
Frankfurter, beef	82.2
Pepperoni	80.8
Avocado	79.5
Walnuts	79.0
Liverwurst	78.5
Bacon (broiled or fried)	77.5
Almonds	75.9
Pork (blade roll, cured)	73.7
Cheese, cheddar	72.5
Peanuts, roasted, salted	71.3

and your blood vessels become less elastic, slowing down your circulation. Imagine, then, being 20, 40 or even 50 pounds overweight. There would be no spring in your step—in fact your knees and ankles would be caving in under the heavy load. The desire to exercise—to move for the joy and pleasure of the movement—would be gone. In fact, it would be a struggle just to rise from a chair.

Overweight, lack of exercise and loss of energy are all related problems that should be considered as one package. As long as the body is forced daily—like one of the slaves who built the pyramids—to relentlessly carry a heavy burden, fatigue is a built-in factor. So it only makes sense that in order to feel more energetic you need to get rid of your excess weight.

CUT CALORIES AS YOU AGE

Overeating can often be a function of not adjusting your caloric intake to your advancing years, says Sheldon Reiser, Ph.D., of the Food and Nutrition Service of the USDA. "We've probably all heard the statement, 'I used to be able to eat everything in sight without gaining weight and now I really have to watch.' As you age, your metabolism slows down so that you need fewer and fewer calories to maintain your body weight," he says.

Middle-aged, sedentary people probably need very few calories to maintain their body weight, says Dr. Reiser. To avoid the energy-robbing habit of overeating, "they should avoid very purified calories that don't supply them the essential nutrients. They'll only have to eat something with nutritious calories afterward." Drinking a 16-ounce cola drink that gives you a generous 160 calories but 40 grams of pure sugar, says Dr. Reiser, is an example of calories not well spent. As you age it's important to milk your calories for the essential nutrients they can give you. After all, vitamins and minerals are the keys that unlock the energy systems of your body.

Of course, exercise, too, helps in a weight-loss program. If you rev

Low-Fat Foods

Low-fat foods should be high on your list when you're trying to control calorie intake. Make foods from this list part of your weight-loss plan.

Food	Percent of Calories from Fat
Apple cider	trace
Raisins, seedless	1.3
Acorn squash	1.5
Peach, fresh	1.8
Bread, Italian	2.0
Grapefruit	2.7
Macaroni, cooked	3.1
Kidney beans, cooked	3.5
Milk, skim	4.5
Turkey breast	4.9
Tuna, canned in water	5.6
Apricots, fresh	6.7
Nectarine	7.7
Butterscotch	8.0
Watermelon	11.3
Oatmeal	13.9
Lobster, broiled	14.2
Gingerbread	20.7

your engine, you'll use more fuel. Step up your activity level and you'll burn more calories. But exercise does more: It leads to energy. Working hard eventually lowers your resting heart rate and your blood pressure, thus relieving your body of an internal burden. Exercise strengthens the muscles and builds endurance. In other words, exercise leads to a normal weight and a fit body. Slim and trim, you'll find yourself dancing—right there in the kitchen!—when your favorite song plays on the radio. And it will no longer be "too much trouble" to run down to the store, or back upstairs to your bedroom, or out to see a friend. Energy. It's never too late to get some. Remember, human energy is a renewable resource.

All this can be yours—but only if you diet properly. The slimmest, trimmest body in the gym isn't going to do you a bit of good if you don't have the stamina to make one lap around the gym.

DIETING AND FATIGUE

Occasionally Jim finds his calorie intake is like supply-side economics—his intake of calories exceeds his energy demands. Yet Jim is resourceful. He usually manages to keep them from turning permanently to fat by working out a little harder at the health club, running a few extra miles and paring unnecessary calories here and there—no sour cream or butter on his potato, no afternoon snacks, smaller dinner and dessert portions. His solution to weight control wasn't always quite so effective. There was a time when Jim, like many of us, tried every fad diet that came along to get rid of his unwanted fat pads.

"A lot of people jump on fad diets," says Art Mollen, D.O., who has guided 10,000 patients to trimmer bodies at his Southwest Health Institute in Phoenix, Arizona. "Many of the fad diets are ultralow in calories," he says. "And, unfortunately, when people are taking perhaps one-quarter of the number of calories that they were used to, they're going to feel a lot of fatigue and a lack of energy. That's because their blood sugar will not stay at a level at which they can function even adequately. Another problem with some diets, even if they have some merit, is that they're not diets that people can stay on forever."

Most of Jim's whimsical dieting was one or another variation on a similar theme: near starvation or drastic reduction in intake of carbohydrates (the supposed bad guys) with no limit on protein. Whether it was "Calories Don't Count" or the "Drinking Man's Diet," the effect was the same. Sure, Jim would lose weight quickly, mostly in the form of fluids. But he would also become incredibly tired and unmotivated to the point where he needed to overeat just to balance his energy economy and feel normal again. It was a vicious cycle as the pounds he worked so hard to lose reaccumulated—just like goods in a free-market glut.

Although many medical authorities have come to recognize the futility of such extreme dieting, each year still seems to bring the latest "miracle diet" with a new twist on the same approach. Yet, as we have seen, the carbohydrates they often severely restrict are some of the best sources of energy. No wonder such diets result in such low energy. Also, unrefined complex carbohydrates such as those in potatoes, rice and whole grain cereals are rich sources of many essential nutrients. Avoid them and you avoid some important energy sparks.

Although it is usually carbohydrates that most fad diets cut out, radically restricting or limiting protein, too, can be just as detrimental to your well-being.

If you accept the premise that we need food to live, then it follows that crash-type dieting can only rob you of the energy to do so. And quick weight loss is almost always followed by quick weight gain—with interest.

THE RIGHT APPROACH

Most of us, like Jim, have the right idea about losing weight, but the wrong approach, especially if we want to maintain the high energy level our workday demands.

The most effective type of diet, energy-wise, as Jim found out, is a sensible one that incorporates exercise and the behavioral changes that help you maintain your normal weight over the long term.

"I see 40 patients a day and they need a diet that's simple, easy and works fast," says Dr. Mollen. "The foods that I recommend for my patients are high-energy complex carbohydrates. I believe that they facilitate a more steady control of the blood sugar instead of quick ups and downs, which are closely linked to fatigue. It's somewhat of a myth that on a high-protein diet you wind up with all kinds of energy, sort of fostered by the image of the football player going out onto the field after eating three steaks. Although protein *is* an essential component in our diet, it is not the direct link to energy. A diet that's high in fat will fatigue you even more easily."

Of course, a total disregard for

calories does not make for a successful diet, says Dr. Mollen. "I put my patients on 1,000, 1,500 or 2,000 calories a day, depending on their weight and what I feel they should lose."

Although carbohydrates are the fastest route to energy in terms of regulating blood sugar during a diet, says Dr. Mollen, this does not mean "you can sit there and eat loads of them and lose weight. You can keep calories down by eating complex carbohydrates in the form of vegetables, salads and some grains. Another old myth was that on a diet you couldn't eat bread, but bread is fine. It's putting 3 tablespoons of mayonnaise or butter on it that creates problems. That's an extra 300 calories!"

WHAT TO EXPECT

When you first begin to diet, even sensibly, the fatigue you may experience is sometimes a psychosomatic effect of the suddenly lowered intake of calories, says Dr. Mollen. "There's a psychological component to recognize here. You feel you're not taking in enough calories so you experience fatigue and a lack of energy." The immediate threat to your diet, says Dr. Mollen, is thinking, "A candy bar is the quick fix I need and I'll feel better."

The smart thing to do, if you want to maintain your diet, your energy and your morale, is to grab a crunchy apple. "You should choose something like this, because the sugar will be absorbed more slowly. You'll have quick absorption of the sugar in the fruit's juice, but then the roughage will cause gradual absorption of the remaining carbohydrate," says Dr. Mollen.

Another advantage to the fiber that most complex carbohydrates are rich in is that it actually seems to help cut calories. A team of researchers at the Veterans' Administration Medical Center in Minneapolis showed this. They fed healthy adults equal amounts of fat in the form of whole peanuts, peanut butter and peanut oil. Less fat was absorbed from the peanuts than from the butter and less from the butter than from the oil. In short, the fiber blocked the absorption of fat and the calories it contains.

Another treat in times of weakening will, says Dr. Mollen, is to take a carrot stick and sprinkle a little sugar substitute on it.

ENERGIZING DIET FOODS

A good diet is also one that gives you the same variety as a nondiet menu. You shouldn't have to look further than your neighborhood supermarket for a variety of diet foods that are also rich in essential nutrients. Put some of these on your shopping list: broccoli and peas (for iron); beets, oranges and romaine lettuce (for folate); beef, chicken, cottage cheese, eggs, yogurt and tuna (for vitamin B_{12}); potatoes, sardines and tomatoes (for potassium); and bananas, brown rice, oatmeal, shredded wheat and spinach (for magnesium).

Dr. Mollen also says, "Although there may be a lot of controversy surrounding taking vitamins and minerals, I think anybody making a switch to a low-calorie diet should certainly take some supplements."

Among the things a good diet should avoid, he says, are caffeine and alcohol. "Caffeine suppresses your appetite by speeding up your central nervous system," says Dr. Mollen. That may seem like a dieter's delight, "but the problem is that your system finally comes back to normal at the end of the day. All of a sudden you're famished, so you eat everything in sight." Dr. Mollen eliminates alcohol from his patients' diets, at least for the first 30 days.

Of course, before you embark on any dramatic change in diet, it's wise to seek personal guidance from your own doctor or a reliable nutritionist.

The secret to maintaining a weight-loss plan and feeling energetic is to find one that you can envision following for the rest of your life, one with rewards. Dr. Mollen recognizes the value of the rewards. His patients who lose their pounds don't get charged for their office visits.

High-Energy Eating

Breakfast—327 Calories
Whole grain muffin
½ cup plain yogurt with 1 cup chopped fruit (apples, oranges, berries), topped with 1 tablespoon chopped walnuts and 1 tablespoon raisins
Herb tea

Lunch—300 Calories
Chunky Chicken-Vegetable Soup
Mixed greens and sprouts salad with 1 tablespoon reduced-calorie vinaigrette dressing
1 slice whole grain bread
1 piece or ½ cup fresh fruit
1 cup decaffeinated coffee

Snack—108 Calories
8 ounces skim milk blended with ½ cup fresh strawberries and ½ teaspoon vanilla extract

Dinner—494 Calories
1 4- to 6-ounce serving Swordfish Vera Cruz
1 cup steamed asparagus or broccoli
1 medium-size baked or steamed potato
Herb tea or grain beverage

Time was when counting calories meant a menu so monotonous it'd bore the life out of your taste buds and take the edge off your energy. Thump! Like a lead weight, right off that diet you'd fall, back to all those forbidden foods. Now we know different. Variety is indeed the indispensable spice of life and moderation is its close ally. Here's a sample 1,200-calorie-a-day menu that proves you can eat nutritious and satisfying low-cal fare without quickly depleting your energy tank. It even includes some of those once blacklisted foods—breads, nuts, dried fruits. They pack a good dose of nutrition and, in *moderate* amounts, add much-needed spunk to your diet.

Chunky Chicken-Vegetable Soup

Makes 6 to 8 servings (106 calories each)

5 cups degreased chicken stock
½ cup diced onion
1 medium leek, diced
1½ cups sliced carrots
½ cup sliced celery
1 clove garlic, minced
1 cup peeled, chopped tomatoes
¼ cup diced sweet pepper
2 tablespoons chopped parsley
½ teaspoon dried thyme
¼ teaspoon dried marjoram
1 tablespoon tamari
1 cup (about ¼ pound) string beans, cut into 1-inch lengths
½ cup peas, fresh or frozen
1¼ cups diced white chicken meat
1 cup diced zucchini
½ cup diced yellow squash
1 cup shredded Swiss chard or spinach

In a large kettle or stock pot, combine stock, onions, leeks, carrots, celery, garlic, tomatoes, peppers, 1 tablespoon parsley, thyme, marjoram and tamari. Bring to a boil over medium heat. Reduce heat to low, cover and simmer 30 minutes. Add string beans. Cover and simmer 10 minutes. Add peas, chicken, zucchini, squash, Swiss chard or spinach and remaining tablespoon of parsley. Continue to simmer 10 minutes longer or until all vegetables are tender.

Swordfish Vera Cruz

Makes 4 servings
(224 calories each)

Fish

    4 cups water
    ¼ cup cider vinegar
    1 bay leaf
    1 lime, sliced
    2 cloves garlic, peeled
    1 allspice berry, crushed
    ¼ teaspoon coriander seeds, crushed
  1⅓ pounds swordfish steak

Sauce

  1½ pounds Italian tomatoes, peeled, seeded and coarsely chopped (about 2 cups), or 1½ 16-ounce cans tomatoes
    3 mild green or serrano chili peppers, seeded and minced, or 1 4-ounce can chili peppers
    1 tablespoon lime juice
    1 tablespoon cider vinegar
    2 tablespoons finely minced onion
    2 cloves garlic, minced
    2 teaspoons dried oregano
    2 allspice berries, crushed
    ½ teaspoon coriander seeds, crushed

To poach the fish, bring the water, vinegar and spices to a boil in a large saucepan. Reduce heat to simmer and add fish. Cover and poach for 15 minutes. Remove from heat and let fish cool in poaching liquid.

While fish is poaching, combine all sauce ingredients in a medium saucepan and bring to a boil.

Reduce heat to low and continue to heat until fish has cooled. Remove fish from poaching liquid and arrange on a platter, then top with sauce and garnish with sliced limes and oranges.

The Fine Art of Snacking

Putting a little creativity into preparation can add to the appeal of nutritious, high-energy snacks. A colorful fruit kabob, a cup of toasty, oil-free popcorn sprinkled with herbs, or a dish of steamed vegetables with yogurt dipping sauce are among the gourmet treats that can complement your dietary needs.

Be creative. Come up with favorites of your own.

3

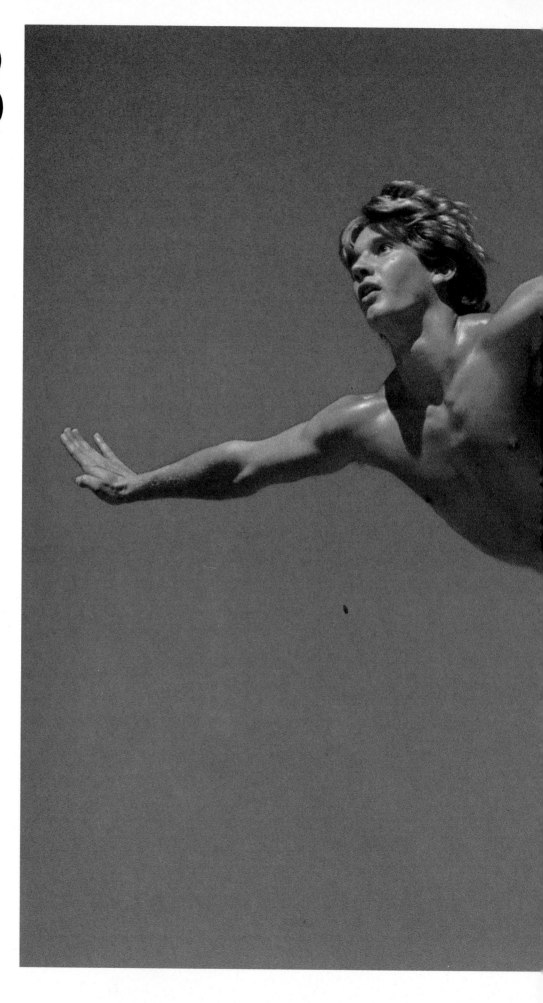

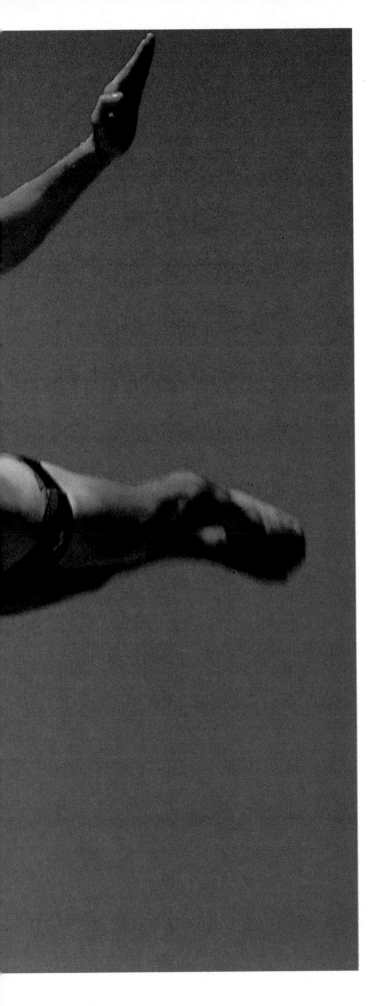

Exercise for Get-Up-and-Go

It's a scientific fact that in order to get energy you must spend energy through an aerobic exercise program.

They call him Dr. Feelgood. He's a wizard at zapping away the blues and the blahs, sculpting dynamic arms and legs, "implanting" stronger hearts and lungs, conjuring up lightning reflexes, instilling superstamina, creating boundless energy and rejuvenating aging bodies. He's even good at soothing frazzled nerves and energizing egos.

The man performs miracles? No. He has just one prescription: exercise!

He works with two easy equations: exercise = energy; energy = good health and fitness.

Dr. Feelgood is a mythical character, but he's really the synthesis of all the physicians and exercise and sports medicine specialists who've been trying to tell us for years that the cure for almost everything that ails us is as simple as regular exercise and sensible nutrition. And the big payoff is *energy*. Energy is exciting, energy is vim and vigor, energy can mean a *new you*.

From the wealth of biomedical and scientific literature available today, it looks like our Dr. Feelgood has been right all along.

Did you know that a National Aeronautics and Space Administration (NASA) study put over 200 federal employees on a not-too-strenuous, regular exercise regimen and came up with some truly fascinating health implications? Ninety percent reported they'd never felt in better health and they had greater stamina; over 60 percent lost weight; almost half of the subjects admitted they felt less stress and tension, they worked harder mentally and physically, enjoyed their jobs more and found their work routines less boring; and almost a third said they slept better.

These people were not born-again fitness buffs; they were ordinary folk who suddenly found

Getting a Foothold on Fitness

You can get a better foothold on exercise with the right shoes. Herman Falsetti, M.D., professor of medicine at the University of Iowa and an adviser to the U.S. Olympic team, recommends softer-soled running shoes to cut down the risk of stress injuries. Ideally, look for air-cushioned soles made of low-density polymer foam with at least 3 layers. A wedge under the heel is also a must. It cuts down wear and tear not only on the foot but also on the body as a whole.

the key to a better life—energy through exercise.

What are you waiting for?

THE OXYGEN CONNECTION

Of course, the type of exercise that's going to do all these wonderful things isn't Tuesday night bowling or Saturday morning golf. Nor is it running five laps around the high school track—every once in a while. It's exercise that keeps you moving—panting good and hard for a good 30 minutes *at least* three times a week. It's what the experts now call aerobic exercise.

Aerobic exercise has swept the nation, yet some may still be puzzled about the magic word *aerobic*. How come this energy-boosting form of fitness didn't spring up and have us bouncing around all over the place a generation ago?

The answer is that we've always been aerobicizing in one way or another. "Aerobics" sounds catchy and cute, so that's probably why the name has caught on and stuck.

Aerobic simply means activity in the presence of oxygen. And that's the secret of aerobic success—utilizing oxygen to provide energy!

To understand why you can't have energy without exercise, let's assume that our human machine is just that—an engine. Its fuel supply is provided by food and oxygen. When we start up the engine it's running at idle, using little gas. Put a foot down on the accelerator (or take off on an exercise routine) and we really start revving. The result is more fuel burned—and that means increased energy.

The more oxygen we feed into our human engine, the more efficiently we metabolize our food. The practical result is that we have more energy.

Unlike a regular engine, our human machine circulates the oxygen that goes into it through the entire body in the bloodstream to reach every cellular level from the tips of our toes to the tiniest gray cell in our brains. It's so efficient that each individual cell in the body is a miniature factory. The cells house the mitochondria, known as the powerhouses of the cell because they are

the sites where energy-supplying ATP is formed.

That's how we can toughen up the heart with aerobic exercise. Even though the heart is a muscle, we don't need to pound and pummel it into shape (although exercising the heart increases strength and overall effectiveness). We can also inject renewed vigor by pumping it full of oxygen.

Bryant Stamford, Ph.D., director of the exercise physiology laboratory at the University of Louisville School of Medicine, explains why our energy quotient depends on aerobic exercise.

First, exercise improves delivery of oxygen to the muscles, says Dr. Stamford. Training increases blood volume and raises the level of oxygen-carrying hemoglobin in red blood cells. The heart becomes capable of pumping greater amounts of blood with each stroke. This also means fewer heartbeats are needed to circulate a given volume of blood, making the heart more work-effective.

Changes also occur in the cells of the skeletal muscles that are involved in the exercise. They now have a greater capacity to use oxygen at the mitochondria level.

With an accelerated delivery and use of oxygen you get increased energy production, which in turn supports muscular contractions for better endurance.

Increased lung volume, enhanced movement of oxygen from the lungs into the blood and the ability to breathe more air per minute all occur with training.

Dr. Stamford says that heart-pumping exercise increases the ability of the muscle cells to use body fat as fuel. At the same time, it preserves valuable glycogen (the stored form of carbohydrates) that serves as the primary source of fuel during heavy exercise. No glycogen, no endurance to go that "extra mile."

Training results in several changes that help prevent heart disease. It melts away unnecessary body fat due to the large number of calories burned, lowers concentrations of cholesterol and triglycerides (blood fats), increases levels of HDL (high-density lipoprotein) cholesterol (the good kind that sweeps fat *away* from the arteries) and reduces high blood pressure.

While all this is going on, the body is becoming tougher: Ligaments that bind bones together at joints become stronger and so do tendons that attach muscles to bone; cartilage, which helps bones fit together at joints, becomes thicker and more durable.

The result: a better-looking, better-feeling, more energized you.

And on top of all this, points out Dr. Stamford, evidence now suggests that aerobic training can improve mental outlook and self-image, reduce tension and anxiety and increase self-discipline, motivation and self-determination.

In fact, a study at the University of Virginia discovered that regular exercise not only improves the body but also energizes the mind, dispels depression and elevates mood.

The key to this remarkable depression-beating strategy was regular exercise programs, not hit-and-miss efforts like playing ball with the boys once or twice a week or the occasional marathon snooker night.

All of the subjects, including those in the study already diagnosed as having recognized clinical depressions, underwent psychological testing to determine their emotional levels. Then they were given exercise choices which ranged from jogging five days a week to playing softball.

At the end of the ten-week trials they were again analyzed for their depressive states.

The results showed that participants who played softball, like those who took no exercise, had unchanged depression levels. Tennis players showed slight but significant mood elevation. The scores for the joggers and the regular exercisers literally bounced up the well-being scale. Even more dramatic was the change in the clinically depressed group of joggers, who were found to exhibit renewed positive outlooks, spontaneous cheerfulness, more energy and increased motivation and activity.

The researchers reported that on this basis "we recommend that any rational, safe and effective treatment for depression should include a prescription for vigorous exercise to bring about and maintain optimal affective functioning."

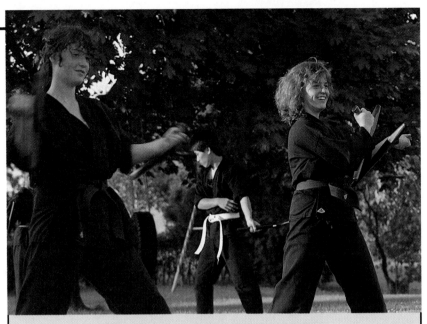

Kids Need Exercise, Too

Kids today are fatter than those in the 1960s, and as many as half of our youngsters may not be getting even enough exercise to develop healthy hearts and lungs. That's the disturbing conclusion of a government study of nearly 9,000 students nationwide. And it doesn't stop there. Fitness skills go hand in hand with better grades, higher self-esteem and good parent/child relationships, reports Charles Kuntzleman, Ed.D., director of the kid-fitness Feelin' Good program. Note to parents: Don't just hug your kids today—get them to exercise, too!

Studies at the University of Montreal, the University of Quebec and Concordia University in Quebec also have confirmed an undeniable link between regular exercise training and higher levels of norepinephrine and prolactin. Fifteen fitness buffs and 15 nonexercisers were subjected to a battery of psychological stress tests. The aerobic group produced more brain antistress chemicals faster, their heartbeats returned to normal more quickly, and they showed less resulting anxiety than their sedentary counterparts. Conclusion: Aerobic-trained individuals may recover faster from stress, both physiologically and emotionally.

The mood and movement connection really does work!

Overtraining

Bill Ruth is an iron man. Give this superathlete a weekly program of 80 to 90 miles of track running and 600 miles of cycling, then throw in 11 miles or so of swimming and he'll tell you this schedule wouldn't faze him one bit.

In fact, this *was* Ruth's grueling workout for the Ironman Triathlon in Hawaii. "I could still have trained harder than that," he says matter-of-factly.

But Ruth burned out.

It can happen to any athlete, just like it can happen to any high-performance machine. You can push only so much, and the biggest fear is that one day it might be too far over the top. When that happens there's only one way to go . . . down! And for most superstars this can often mean the finish line as far as future competition goes.

"Top athletes are always on the borderline of overtraining," points out E. C. Frederick, Ph.D., director of research for Nike, Inc. "Much of the time it's very deliberate. Coaches use the technique to take them over the edge and bring them back." They get what's called rebound phenomena— added strength and endurance. "But I've seen it backfire, even among Olympic-caliber athletes," he says.

To create peak performance, according to the training specialists, the body has to be stretched to its limits. What they don't like to admit is that this means the human condition is literally torn down just so that it can be rebuilt—mostly in the exact image the coach desires. Blood vessels, tissue, tendons and muscles can't escape damage as they go through the grinder in pursuit of future athletic perfection.

And Dr. Frederick warns that ordinary exercise enthusiasts can be at even greater risk than the carefully monitored pros.

"Most beginners have an encounter with overtraining early on; it's also the reason why many give up on exercise. You see them—they're the ones with tendonitis, the characters with shinsplints. It's simply the result of too much, too soon," warns Dr. Frederick.

Dr. Bryant Stamford of the University of Louisville School of Medicine blames the overtraining problem on a few well-held myths among athletes and exercise novices, those who proclaim, "The harder you practice, the better you'll play," and "No pain, no gain!"

Bill Ruth found out the hard way. While in sixth place in the Ironman competition, he collapsed from dehydration and had to drop out. Also, his hamstrings, which had flared up before the race, got worse and he had a backbreaking schedule of other competitions. Portland, Oregon, saw him develop blisters on his feet; outside Philadephia he crashed his bike and injured a shoulder. In July and August he had six races in six weeks and each time he felt more like death. He developed boils on his arms and thighs. Eventually he couldn't get out of bed.

How do you know if you're overtraining? Here are some symptoms:

- You crawl out of today's exercise and loathe the thought of tomorrow's.
- You have trouble sleeping.
- You have no energy to enjoy doing other things.
- Your morning pulse rate is high.
- Your appetite is out of control or you have no appetite at all.
- You begin to develop aches and pains you never had before.

Here's what to do:

- Listen to your body. If it feels bad, it's trying to tell you something.
- Rest up. Most exercise physiologists recommend this as your first and most valuable line of defense, and by far the best cure. Just taking a day or two away from your regular exercise program can do the trick.
- Massages, saunas and gentle manipulative exercises can help. So can certain muscle relaxants and anti-inflammatory drugs, including aspirin.
- Try taking on an additional, less taxing exercise or sport. It's refreshing, not only psychologically but physiologically.

Alberto Salazar's Dramatic Story

Marathon runners are caught in an ironic dilemma. The extreme physical demands of their sport force them to undertrain. The drive to win tempts them to overtrain. Confused? Now you know how they feel.

The human body refuses to allow marathoners to run the devastating 26-mile races in practice. "The reason is, nobody could take it," says Alberto Salazar, former holder of the world record (2:08.13). "The limit is about 20 miles a day in two separate sets." In contrast, boxers sometimes spar 20 rounds per session to get ready for a 15-round fight. Football players, basketball stars, swimmers, sprinters and medium-distance runners all train up to, or more than, the less draining time period or distance of their sport. Marathoners have no such guidelines. Therein lies the endless problem—how much, or how little, should they run?

"The majority of long-distance runners overtrain," admits Salazar, a Boston Marathon champion and 3-time winner of the New York Marathon. "The tendency is to push on, to run that extra mile or two, trying to find that extra edge, that optimum level. When you get lucky and hit upon the right level for you, that's when you run your best times. When you overdo it, you begin to feel stale in workouts. The energy just isn't there. It can affect your sleep, your mood, performance, every-thing. Overtraining is something we are constantly fighting."

It's a fight Salazar admits he's recently lost. Once virtually unbeatable, his performance plunged so drastically in 1983 that he finished dead last in the 10,000 meters at the Helsinki games. At the 1984 Olympics, he finished 14th in the marathon, a race he had once been favored to win. He went, as they say, from the penthouse to the outhouse. Three things did Salazar in—injuries, his fierce training schedule and a deficiency in iron resulting in fatigue similar to that suffered by anemics. (Thanks to Salazar, iron loss was discovered to be a common problem among long-distance runners.)

Surprisingly, part of the problem turned out to be that the vital iron was being pounded into use-lessness by constant run-ning. Blood cells in his feet were smashed, their iron lost. "I've been taking iron supplements, and it's helped," Salazar said. "I've also cut down on my running, from 130 miles a week to about 100. I just tried to train and race at too high a level for too long a time. It caught up with me. The thing to remember is you can run better undertrained than flirting with disaster and being overtrained."

Take Five to Energize

Low on gusto? Can't seem to get moving? Here's a 5-minute energizer designed to zap you back into action. These 10 exercises are simple to do and can be done anywhere, anytime.

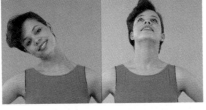

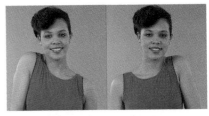

1 **Head Rolls.** Start with your feet a little more than shoulder width apart and turned out slightly. Using a count of 4, let your head fall forward like a dead weight, then left, then back, then right. Perform the sequence twice.

2 **Shoulder Lifts.** Shrug your shoulder, then push it down. Do 5 times with each shoulder.

6 **Long Legs.** When you've completed the last windmill, stay bent over. Bend your knees and put your palms flat on the floor between and slightly in front of your feet. Look up and in front of you. Now lower your head and straighten your legs.

7 **Reach-Outs.** With your feet spread, turn your body toward your left leg. Point your left foot to the left and turn your right foot perpendicular to your left heel. Extend your arms in front of you and reach out like a sleepwalker, stretching forward, then back. Your left leg bends, your right stays straight. Do 10 times in each direction.

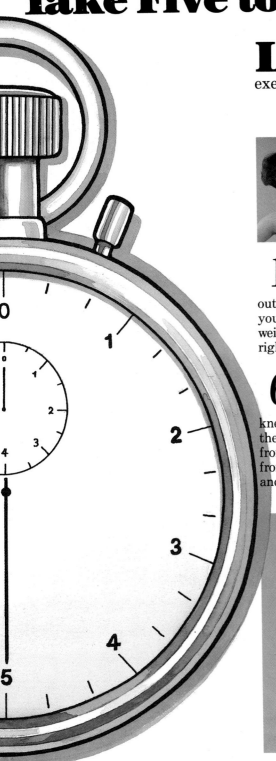

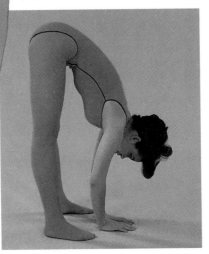

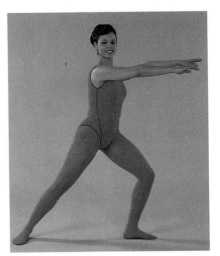

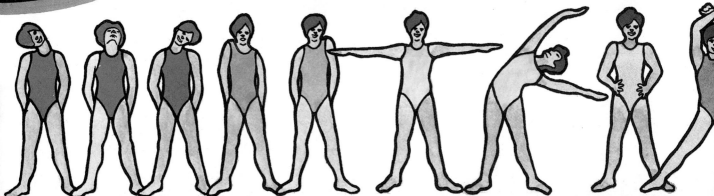

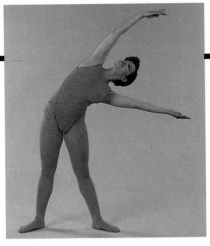
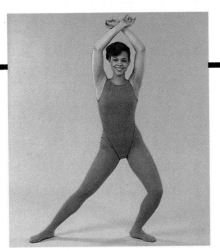
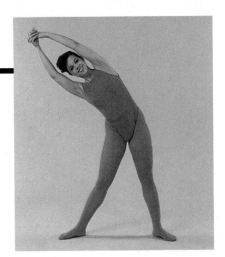

3 **Waist Stretches.** Extend your arms to the sides at shoulder level. Bending at the waist, stretch to the left, bringing your right arm up and over your head. Look straight up at your palm and count to 4, then return to center. Repeat to the right side, counting to 4. Then do 5 times quickly on each side without counting.

4 **Inner Thigh Stretches.** Stand with your feet spread, hands on hips. Now lean left, bending your left leg but keeping your right leg straight, while you reach up and cross your wrists over your head. Return to center, bringing your hands back to your hips. Do 5 times on each side.

5 **Windmills.** Bend forward from the waist, lacing your fingers together near the floor. Now swing your upper body erect to the right, then down to the left, making a complete circle. Do 5 times in each direction.

8 **Jazz Stretch.** Bring your feet together and slowly bend over. Grab your ankles or calves and *gently* pull your head toward your knees. Breathe deeply and hold for a count of 4. Now slowly unbend.

9 **Jog in Place.** Lift those heels up and swing those arms! Think of yourself as a golden retriever let loose in an endless meadow. Jog for a count of 50.

10 **Forward Kicks.** Keep jogging, kicking your right foot forward with a small kick and pushing forward with your left arm. Then kick with your left foot and push with your right arm. Try to be fluid, and keep it up for a count of 50.

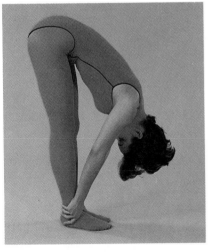
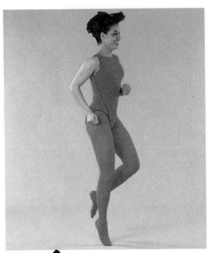
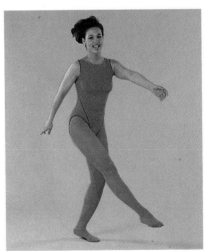

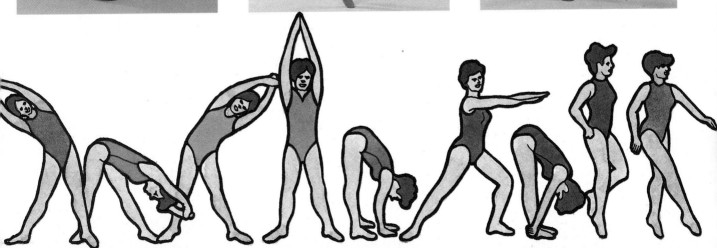

Rating the Energy Supplements

Performance boosting! That's the name of the game for many professional and weekend athletes alike. To help things along, some athletes use "ergogenic aids," or more simply, nutrients, foods or formulas that are purported to give extra energy. These substances range from straightforward vitamins and minerals to odd items like bee pollen. Recent surveys show that up to 80 percent of athletes take such supplements for training and competition. But do they really work? Let's find out what the experts say.

Amino Acids and Protein Powders. It seems like a smart move—the body uses amino acids to build protein, and protein builds muscles, so take amino acids or protein powder (a concentrated source, usually from animal tissue), and you'll have bigger (and maybe stronger) muscles. Only it doesn't quite work out that way. All that extra protein doesn't build muscle (if it did, every burger lover would have bulging biceps). Only exercise can do that—stressed muscles break down and then repair, getting bigger in the process. So where does the extra protein go? A lot of it is excreted, and in the process it breaks down into substances that tax the kidneys and may even *cause* fatigue. Not exactly what an ergogenic aid is supposed to do!

But the protein press isn't all bad. One amino acid, leucine, can shore up ailing muscle tissue in postsurgical patients. Will it help postinjury athletes? It's too early to tell.

And some competitors—particularly body builders who want to look like Charles Atlas clones—may need more protein than us mortals. But is protein powder—which usually has a price tag that makes you think the label should read "platinum powder" —the way to get it?

"I tell athletes, instead of going out and paying outrageous prices for amino acids and protein powders, go to the local grocery store and buy powdered milk instead," says William J. Evans, Ph.D., chief of the Physiol-

ogy Laboratory of the Human Nutrition Research Center at Tufts University. "It's a very high-quality protein at one-twentieth the cost, and it's low in fat and cholesterol."

Vitamin B$_6$ (Pyridoxine). Like protein, B$_6$ looks good in *theory*. That's because B$_6$ is crucial in breaking down glycogen (stored body fuel) to liberate instant energy. But a word of warning here: Studies on B$_6$ boosting have shown that a too-rapid breakdown of glycogen can lead to early exhaustion —and that's just the opposite of what you're trying to achieve.

That's the conclusion from research conducted among athletes at Oregon State University. James Lecklem, Ph.D., associate professor of foods and nutrition at the university, who reviewed the test findings on B$_6$, warns, "I feel athletes should be cautious here."

Glucose and Fructose. These two sugars are often included in "high-energy" drinks and work on the premise that by supplying additional sugars, you can replace the glycogen burned up by exercise.

There's no doubt that this works, but the effects appear to be minimal—a "quick fix" at most. Over the long haul—like a marathon or an all-day tournament—it may actually accelerate rather than decrease muscle fatigue.

And it seems that glucose works but fructose doesn't. In a recent study comparing the fatigue-delaying power of glucose or fructose to that of water, glucose delayed exhaustion from heavy exercise by 20 percent. Fructose did nothing.

Thiamine (Vitamin B$_1$). If you know anybody who's taking thiamine for energy, you can tell them they're living in the sports nutrition Dark Ages. No studies have shown any energy-boosting effects from additional thiamine, only that *deficiencies* can contribute to fatigue. We get sufficient levels through our normal diet.

This nutrient got its best press after the 1939 Tour de France when it was used by the winners, but decades went by with no further evidence to substantiate its benefits. Even the most up-to-date research on this nutrient was wrapped up almost 20 years ago.

Riboflavin (Vitamin B₂). A study in Quebec of eight male and six female swimmers, ranked among Canada's top ten, looked at riboflavin versus placebos (fake pills that look like the real thing). When the aquatic elite were put to the test in six freestyle bouts of 50 meters each, then on treadmills to the point of exhaustion, no difference was found between those who took the riboflavin and the ones who took the placebos.

Vitamin C. An Israeli study of 33 sedentary males given either 1,000 milligrams of vitamin C or a placebo, then trained in running and hiking, showed no differences between the two groups. Worse still, an Alabama study of 15 healthy men, who were given 600 milligrams of C or a placebo and then tested for maximum endurance, showed the placebo group did better! Vitamin C won't give competitors the winning edge.

Vitamin E. Some athletes swear by it for endurance and lungs that just won't quit.

There's actually little or no evidence to link E to the metabolic processes of energy. But where the lungs are concerned, there may be actual benefit. The vitamin is recognized as a powerful antioxidant, and its actions may help in warding off the effects of air pollution—a very significant factor, for example, if you're running the New York or Boston marathon, or even just jogging around town.

Another study also indicates a connection between vitamin E and the lungs. Supplementation with E at high altitudes (5,000 to 15,000 feet) seemed to increase aerobic capacity.

Octacosanol. It's an active ingredient in wheat germ oil, and it's garnered the endorsements of such sporting luminaries as tennis ace Martina Navratilova.

Its biggest promoter is Thomas K. Cureton, Ph.D., of the University of Illinois, who's spent 20 years in studies that claim to show increased endurance and stamina and extra vigor among athletes.

But it's not without critics. After reviewing Dr. Cureton's work, Melvin Williams, Ph.D. director of the human performance lab at Old Dominion University in Virginia, says categorically that there's not one valid study to provide any reasons for taking octacosanol.

The Truth about Electrolyte Drinks

Just the sound of the name "electrolyte drink" gives a wonderful mental picture of a chock-full-of-nutrients drink zapping you full of instant energy and getting you over the finish line—first.

The truth is that electrolyte drinks (or sports drinks)—which contain sugar and nutrients such as magnesium, potassium and sodium—have little if anything to do with improving performance. For one thing, an athlete doesn't lose enough electrolytes during a workout to require replenishing. The human performance lab at Ball State University in Indiana reports that the body is so marvelously self-regulating that you must push yourself to superhuman limits to deplete its electrolyte stockpile.

Also, these drinks actually have a handicap. Because they contain sugar and concentrated amounts of electrolytes, the stomach empties slower, meaning it takes longer for the nutrients to get to the bloodstream where they are needed.

The verdict? For ordinary, daily exercise training, electrolyte beverages are not necessary, says William Fink, assistant to the director of the Ball State lab. They won't harm you, but neither will they improve your performance. Just remember to drink plenty of *water* to replace any excess fluid loss.

4

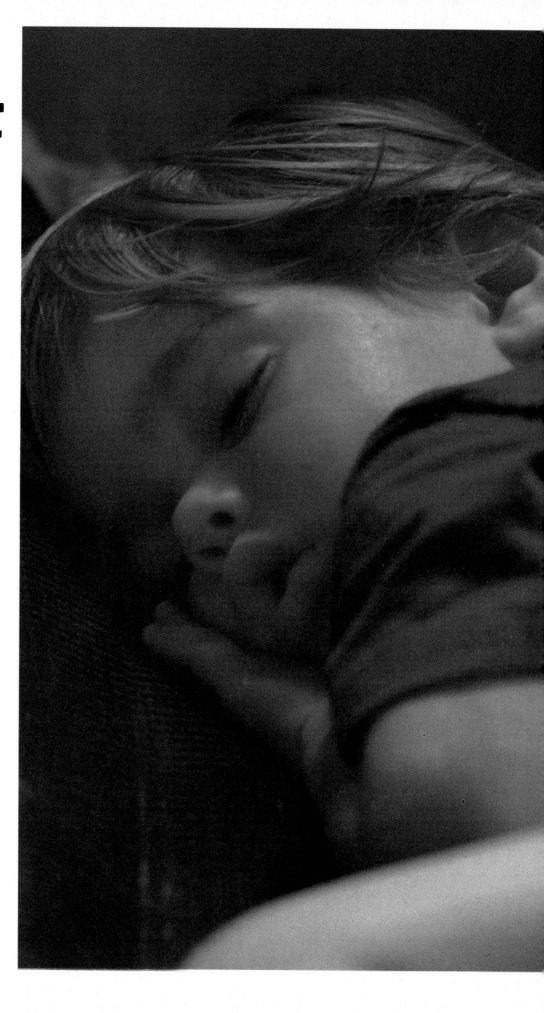

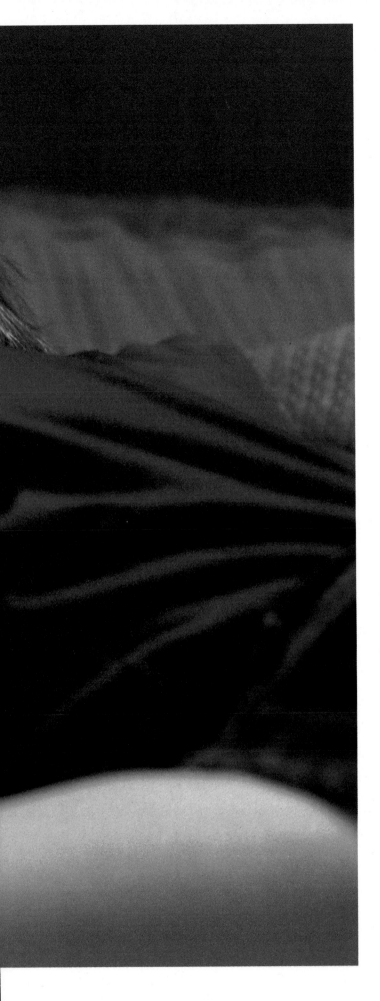

Sleep: The Quiet Energizer

Understand the importance of satisfying slumber and your life will take on new zest.

There is nothing that refreshes the body and the mind quite like a good night's sleep. You crawl bone-weary into bed at night, then reawaken the next day full of pep and enthusiasm, ready and eager to face a whole new day of challenging activities.

At least that's the way it's supposed to work. Unfortunately, sleep—the most powerful and easily identified of the natural energy boosters—is a complicated, oftimes elusive commodity that is only now getting the careful and intensive research that it so richly deserves.

Surprisingly, up until about 35 years ago sleep was pretty much an unknown quantity. Everybody understood its value, of course, but nobody understood just how it worked. Now, as sleep researchers carefully observe people at rest and chart the changes that occur in their bodies during slumber, they are able not only to help improve the energizing quality of this all-important activity but also to counsel and help those millions for whom sleep is so difficult to obtain.

Perhaps the most important cornerstone in the understanding of sleep was the discovery that we function on what scientists call circadian rhythms. These rhythms oscillate on approximately 25-hour cycles and regulate more than 100 biological activities on a continuing basis. Our temperature, respiration, mood, alertness and hormone secretions all rise and fall at approximately the same time within the cycle. Scientists have determined that for the majority of people— the "day" folks among us—temperatures generally peak in the morning and are at their lowest during the night. It should come as no surprise, then, to learn that we function at our best when our temperatures are highest and at our worst when they are lowest.

Just as you might have suspected, it is during

our waking hours—our time of activity and movement—that our body tissues break down. During our waking hours, our bodies also pump great amounts of adrenaline—that all-important hormone that keeps us responding effectively to emergencies. But adrenaline inhibits the formation of the protein that is needed to repair the normal wear and tear our tissues go through every day. And this is why sleep's so important. Only during sleep does the flow of adrenaline stop almost completely. This allows the growth hormone secreted by the pituitary gland to kick into action and renew our weary tissues. In other words, we literally burn up tissue during the day and renew it at night while we sleep.

Wakefulness = energy. Rest = renewal. It all sounds so natural, so attainable. But unfortunately, it's not. To everyone's occasional dismay, and to an alarming number of people's continuing distress, it is not always possible to get the amount of sleep our bodies require. Sleep researchers estimate that energy-robbing insomnia affects as much as one-third of the adult population during the course of a year. And an estimated 20 to 25 million people suffer from disturbed sleep night after night. It's no wonder so many people seem to start their day as if they got up on the wrong side of the bed!

THE FIVE FACES OF INSOMNIA

There are many causes of insomnia, and they can range from the simple physical pain of a stubbed toe to deep-rooted psychological problems. Environment, too, is important, as evidenced by the increased incidence of sleeplessness in crowded, noisy cities. Needless to say, since there is no one cause of insomnia, there is no one cure.

Alice K. Schwartz, Ph.D., a psychologist, and Norma S. Aaron, Ph.D., a psychological consultant, both members of the American Psychological Association, have done extensive research into insomnia. They've divided it into five classifications—each with its own prescribed cure. The five classifications have complicated, scientific-sounding names, but they describe conditions easily identified by people who have trouble sleeping. Finding the category that fits you, they believe, is the first step in battling your insomnia. Here are the five.

Initardia. This is the inability to fall asleep, a common condition probably most often identified with the term insomnia.

Hyperlixia. This term describes an excessive amount of light sleep. It is a form of insomnia that often goes unrecognized because many of its victims believe they have spent the whole time awake.

Pleisomnia. This type of insomnia is characterized by sleep interrupted by frequent awakenings. It often appears after the age of 40.

Scurzomnia. This condition is short sleep, in which a person falls asleep easily and sleeps well. After a couple of hours, however, the insomniac

---

Say No to the Nightcap

It's been one of those days, the kind when you jump out of bed and hit the floor running, never really to catch up or even get a moment's relaxation. Now the hour is getting late and you're too tense, too keyed-up to even think of falling asleep.

The answer, millions believe, is a couple of drinks to turn those rough edges smooth and bring on the rest that will help you cope with the rigors of tomorrow.

Trouble is, the answer is wrong.

What happens, explains Michael Stevenson, Ph.D., director of the insomnia clinic at Holy Cross Hospital, Mission Hills, California, is this: "About 2 to 3 hours after drinking you go through alcohol withdrawal, which actually arouses the nervous system to a higher level than before . . . If the wine is at bedtime, you may fall asleep easily, only to find yourself wide awake in the middle of the night."

A rule to remember: Alcohol induces sleep, but it interferes with rest.

awakens and is unable to return to sleep.

Turbula. This is troubled sleep, the kind interrupted by frequent nightmares. This problem is most often associated with personal unhappiness and stress.

HELP FOR THE WORRIERS

Initardia is often the result of an erratic lifestyle, the kind in which pressure-packed days make a shambles of a healthy routine. Tension can crop up at any time, meals are often on the run or late in the evening, and the worries of the day often crawl right into bed with the victims of sleeplessness.

To counteract the effects of this typically modern way of living, Dr. Schwartz and Dr. Aaron recommend first that a person develop a presleep routine—opening the window, brushing teeth, putting on nightclothes, setting the alarm, etc. —and follow it each night. The value of this set routine is that it will help remind the mind that sleep is to follow. The researchers even have found that you can help yourself to fall asleep by reminding yourself consciously that "I will fall asleep more quickly tonight."

They also suggest that a healthier sleep pattern can be encouraged by going to bed at the same time every night and setting the alarm (and getting up!) an hour earlier than normal. This should help to induce fatigue, and sleep, on subsequent nights. After sleep starts to come more easily, the alarm can be gradually moved back to your normal wake-up time.

Not to be forgotten, either, is the value of exercise. A properly developed exercise program can help slumber come more easily.

DON'T BE A SLEEPYHEAD!

With hyperlixia, researchers have found the problem may actually be one of too much sleep. While the victims may believe they are getting no sleep at all, they are actually nodding off so often, day and night,

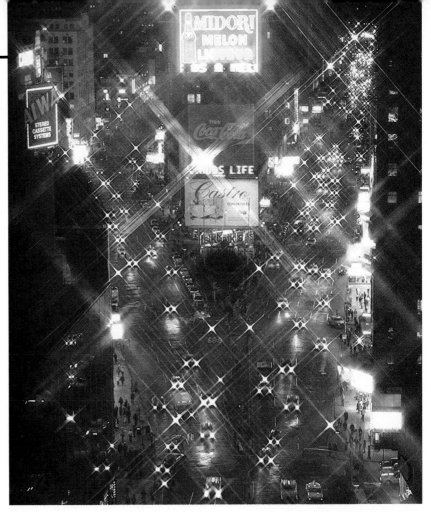

that they are incapable of getting that restorative deep sleep at their normal bedtime. As a first step in eliminating the problem, these insomniacs are advised to carefully chart all the time spent lying down each day, all the time spent relaxing on the sofa or the chaise lounge, and all the time spent dozing while seated. If all those periods add up to an adequate amount of sleep time, but they still feel uncomfortable about night sleep, they probably have hyperlixia.

As with most problems involving sleeplessness, the most obvious cure is to make sure that you go to bed tired. (A regular program of sustained exercise can help here, too.)

When you awaken at night, you should look at the clock. If you find that big chunks of unexplained time keep passing, you can be assured that you actually have been sleeping lightly. The only task then is to convince yourself that you're getting decent rest—perhaps by the simple method of actually telling yourself, "I must have been asleep. I must have been sleeping." When that

For many people, the neverending hustle and bustle of a major metropolitan area contribute to a rich and exciting personal life. Unfortunately, for many others that same tense, noisy and competitive atmosphere often contributes to one of the major irritants of big-city life—insomnia.

happens, deeper, more satisfying sleep should follow.

MAKE YOURSELF TIRED

Pleisomnia—sleep characterized by frequent awakenings—can be traced to a variety of causes. In order to guarantee that sleep is consolidated in one uninterrupted block, the first thing to do is create a situation in which the body is crying out for rest.

The best way to achieve this is simply to force yourself to sleep less. Start by going to bed an hour later than usual, taking care to wake up at your normal time. If that doesn't do the job, set your bedtime back an hour and a half—or even more, if necessary. The important thing is to go to bed so weary that the body will automatically repel any desire to stay awake. It also might be helpful to alter the bedroom atmosphere. You can change the decorations and fur-

Four Ways to Feel Fine after Four Hours (or Less) of Sleep

The error of your ways becomes apparent as soon as you hear the alarm clock. Even as you are reaching over to shut the darned thing off you can sense the deep grogginess, the burning eyes that have not yet been opened.

Slowly it all comes back to you. The person who gave you "a book that you just can't put down" was right. Now you are about to start a new day preceded by just a few hours of sleep—*too few* hours of sleep. You will definitely rise, but it doesn't seem likely that you will shine.

Most of us have had similar experiences, probably more often than we care to admit, and have dreaded the thought of dragging ourselves through a day listless and drained of natural energy.

Well, it doesn't have to be that way. By following a few commonsense tips, you really can minimize the problems brought on by an occasional slip in your normal sleep routine.

One of the best remedies is also the most obvious. "If possible, try and work in a nap," advises Elliott R. Phillips, M.D., medical director of the sleep disorders center at Holy Cross Hospital in Mission Hills, California, and author of *Get a Good Night's Sleep*. "A lot of people can be refreshed after as few as 20 minutes of sleep." (Of course, naps are not advisable for those people who find

themselves even more drowsy afterward or for sufferers of chronic insomnia.)

But for those who cannot make time for 40 winks, there are other methods. "The more active you are, the easier it will be to get through the day," he says. "For some people a period of exercise will be as good as a nap. . . . In addition, animal studies suggest that disruptions in your exercise routine may upset your sleep patterns."

Another important aid is to make sure you get up as close as possible to your normal waking time—even if it is Saturday morning and you have nothing pressing to do. Our bodies are kept in sync by our circadian rhythms. The lack of sleep obviously disturbs the rhythm. By getting up at your usual time you at least will not be perpetuating the disturbance. It also is important, for the same reason, to maintain a regular eating pattern.

For some people, the temporary use of stimulants such as coffee or tea may be appropriate. But take care not to overuse the beverages, because too much caffeine can disrupt sleep later on.

Dr. Phillips notes that these tips are useful only for occasional sleepless nights. They're no cure for abuse night after night.

nishings in your bedroom to make your surroundings more pleasant. There is nothing wrong with leaving a night light lit if you find it helps to make you feel more relaxed.

Sometimes, pleisomnia is caused by mental anguish. It might pay to do a little soul searching to determine any underlying depression, anxiety, fear or anger that may be causing the problem. Often, these psychological factors can be diminished or eliminated by a daily regimen of vigorous exercise, so long as the exercise is done during the day. (Exercise at bedtime will only keep you awake.)

GOT THE FIDGETS?

To people with an active, vigorous lifestyle, scurzomnia might at first seem to be something of a blessing. You fall asleep easily, rest well, and after only a few hours you feel rested and raring to go. Great? Well, not really. For people with this problem, that ready-for-anything spunk fades fast. Fatigue can set in when energy hasn't even peaked in those who naturally can get by on little sleep. Drowsiness, aching muscles and burning eyes occur when you really should be alert and efficient.

Exercise—vigorous and in periods from an uninterrupted 30 minutes to an hour or more—is a particularly helpful antidote to scurzomnia. This shouldn't be asking too much, since scurzomniacs are usually active to begin with. Just remember, no exercise at night! The key is to induce muscle fatigue, so a leisurely stroll or housework will not qualify.

Another way to alleviate the problem is to shorten potential sleep time. Try going to bed one hour later than usual. If you find this difficult (late-night talk shows may just not be stimulating enough), plan active projects for your evening, activities that stimulate your small muscles as well as your mind. Examples are sewing, cooking, woodworking and painting. Naps should be avoided at all costs: Persons prone to scurzomnia should make sure they do not even lie down during the day. Like any other bad sleeping habit, scurzomnia can be defeated by altering habit patterns.

ENDING UGLY NIGHTMARES

Turbula, sleep characterized by unpleasant dreams and nightmares, often follows a personal loss or an unpleasant and unhappy personal situation. The dreams can be considered expressions of grief. Generally, the sleep problem will subside as the trouble that caused it fades into the recesses of the mind.

Surprising as it may seem, it is possible for people to avoid the terror of nightmares by learning to wake themselves up before the dreams build in intensity. What is involved is a bit of self-hypnosis, the same kind people use in acquiring the ability to awaken at a particular time. (How many people do you know who claim they don't need an alarm clock?)

All you must do is tell yourself you must awaken as soon as a nightmare begins. While this may sound difficult, researchers have found that the decision alone, with no further instructions, is usually all that's required to make it work.

It is also helpful to bring into focus the circumstances of your nightmares. Try to picture the setting, think about the people involved, recall the noises that accompany the dream, review and try to feel the emotions you experienced. In short, you can train yourself, through reexamination of your dreams, to identify the warning signals of an impending nightmare.

It is important, too, not to fall right back to sleep after an unpleasant dream episode. Get out of bed and go sit in a chair, preferably in another room. Then, for 5 minutes, stroke your right forearm with your left fingertips. According to Dr. Schwartz and Dr. Aaron, this exercise is designed to interfere with and terminate the agitation of nerves that accompanies nightmares. It will disrupt the neural patterns that accompany the troubled sleep.

THE BIG SLEEP

The researchers also have uncovered evidence that there may be one factor that for some is an underlying cause of all forms of insomnia—fear of death. This type of insomnia affects people who equate sleep with death. To them, fear of death translates into fear of sleep.

If you are wondering if this might be your problem, ask yourself these questions: Do you wake up with a start, feeling instantly alert? Many people who are fearful of death experience this. Are you afraid of the dark? If not now, have you ever been? Death and darkness are also associated with each other. If you were faced with an operation, would you prefer a local anesthetic or one that puts you to sleep? The correlation here is obvious. Is your sleep problem related to the recent death of a friend or relative? Such grievous incidents in our lives can trigger the death fear in us.

If you have determined to your own satisfaction that your sleep problems are associated with a fear of death, the researchers suggest that you begin building new habit patterns that will make sleep become an inviting and enjoyable activity. You can give yourself a little extra luxury at bedtime (a nice snack, for instance) and, if possible, engage in sexual activity. The association of sleep with pleasure will reduce its association with death.

THE KNACK OF NAPPING

For many thousands of people, sleep almost never comes in one satisfying and rejuvenating nighttime package. These are the nappers, the people who find it necessary to grab 40 winks now and then.

But is napping good for your health? Is it an effective energy booster? Does it really make you more efficient? What actually happens when you take a nap?

One study that attempted to answer those questions was conducted at the Institute of Pennsylvania Hospital in Philadelphia and involved 430 college students. It identified three different kinds of nappers: those who nap only to make up for lost sleep, those who nap because they derive a psychological benefit, and those who nap in response to stress-induced insomnia. This last sort of sleep,

researchers noted, "is not satisfying and tends to interfere with the subsequent night's sleep"—meaning that a sleep disturbance resulted in the need for a nap.

There is still another group, they point out: nonnappers for whom "the aftermath of napping seems to be sufficiently unpleasant that it is to be actively avoided." The study indicates that one important difference between nappers and nonnappers is that nappers have far more voluntary control over sleep because they are able to fall asleep easily almost anywhere.

After monitoring each group during 60-minute naps in the sleep lab, the researchers discovered that the so-called replacement nappers descended into deep sleep in much the same way night sleepers do. So did most of those who considered themselves nonnappers. But those who napped only because they enjoyed it slept quite differently, fluctuating between drowsiness and several levels of light sleep. They later reported experiencing states of dreamlike reverie.

"Some people have the capacity to nap as needed to compensate for accumulated sleep deficits; others use the nap primarily for psychological restorative functions seemingly unrelated to sleep needs," the researchers concluded.

Another study, conducted at Ohio State University, indicated that merely lying down and resting may be as beneficial as actually falling asleep. In the study, 20 habitual nappers were monitored during a 1-hour nap in the laboratory, as were 20 others who were asked to rest in bed without falling asleep.

The subjects were given a series of performance tests and asked to report on their mood before and after the experiment. The nappers slept 61 percent of the time, the nonnappers not at all. And although both groups improved significantly in mood and performance, neither group outdid the other.

WHO SHOULD TAKE NAPS?

So who should take naps? Who shouldn't? If you find a nap truly refreshing and it doesn't interfere with your sleep at night, then please, nap to your heart's content. But if you suffer from insomnia or you are an elderly person who has trouble falling asleep at night, you should avoid naps entirely or, at the very least, nap at the same time each day. "If you want to improve nighttime sleeping, don't take a sometime nap," cautions Quentin Regestein, M.D., director of the sleep clinic at Boston Brigham and Women's Hospital.

The length of naps depends on individual needs. "Moderation is the key," warns John M. Taub, Ph.D., a sleep researcher in St. Louis. "Just as oversleeping can make you feel groggy, when I 'overnap,' I feel terrible."

Dr. Taub also says that there is no ideal time for napping. The most beneficial time for napping depends on an individual's biological clock.

The need for and benefits of napping, the studies show, seem to vary from person to person. If a nap doesn't work for you, just don't do it. If it does, by all means enjoy it.

After all, one research team has noted that the refreshing results of a short snooze "seem to have restorative value far exceeding the length of time involved."

SOME SLEEP TOO MUCH

Unfortunately for some, a short snooze in the afternoon has no restorative value at all. In fact, it sometimes only leads to another nap—a vicious cycle that leaves you groggy and lethargic. This could mean your problem is more serious than needing a little rest.

Excessive sleepiness during the day, the inability to stop napping, or taking naps that do not seem to refresh you could mean that you are suffering from a sleep disorder.

One such condition is known as sleep apnea, in which sleep is interrupted hundreds of times due to unexplained cessation of breathing. Sufferers tend to be overweight and usually snore heavily. Those who suffer from a condition called nocturnal myoclonus are also wakened repeatedly during the night, but because of involuntary leg jerking. Usually, those with either disorder

(continued on page 54)

Famous Nappers

Salvador Dali did it with a spoon in his hand, John Kennedy did it in his pajamas, and Thomas Edison used to do it on the laboratory couch. It is a nap, that revitalizing respite that can turn pooped into peppy, those 40 winks that can turn the weary into winners.

Stress-filled world leaders, famous artists and entertainers, scientists and business tycoons— they've all been caught napping from time to time. And, for the most part, they are outspoken advocates of the practice.

Obviously, not everyone is as inventive as the great Spanish surrealist, Dali. He reportedly dozed off while holding a spoon in his hand over a metal plate. When the spoon fell from his hand onto the plate, the noise awakened him. Kennedy, his associates reported, preferred to get into his night-clothes and climb into bed for his frequent 45-minute afternoon naps. The inventor Edison is credited with a long and creative life that included 4 hours or less of sleep a night. But it was later established that he managed this only by taking frequent naps in the laboratory whenever his mind became weary.

Those are but a few of the famous nappers, part of a list that includes such luminaries as presidents Johnson and Truman, Sir Winston Churchill, Napoleon, Mayor Ed Koch of New York, Eleanor Roosevelt and Malcolm Forbes.

If there is one thing all these people have in common, it is that their lives defy normal routine. The nap appears to be one thing which helps solve the problems of a tiring and erratic lifestyle.

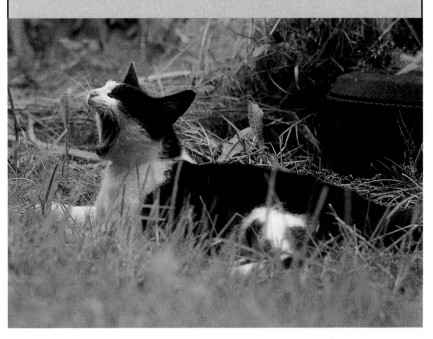

The Problem of Shift Work

In the best of all possible worlds, the majority of us probably would turn out to be day people. We would awaken without alarm clocks and go about our business vigorously until, sometime after dark, we would begin to feel heavy with fatigue and retire for the night. We would be healthy and energetic, our bodies fully replenished each night to face the rigors of the succeeding day.

We know this to be true because we all have built-in "biological clocks" —wake/sleep cycles that correspond with the hours of light and darkness.

The problem is that many of us don't live in the best of all possible worlds. Millions of us have schedules that are determined not by our biological clocks but by the demands of modern society in which we manufacture goods around the clock, require 24-hour police protection and medical care, travel across time zones and generally cram more activity into a 24-hour day than nature ever intended.

Charles A. Czeisler, M.D., Ph.D., of Harvard Medical School and Boston Brigham and Women's Hospital, cites statistics that show that one out of every four working men and one of every six working women—20 to 30 million people—have a variable work schedule that throws their "clocks" out of whack. They're yearning for breakfast when everyone else is eating dinner, or climbing into bed after a hard night's work just as the daily traffic jam is forming outside their windows.

The results of this disruption are predictable. Millions stumble through their daily (or nightly) lives listlessly, operating inefficiently and feeling rotten because of the unnatural lifestyles forced upon them by their jobs or their personal lifestyles. Worse yet, an erratic life can be downright dangerous.

Truck accidents, for example, are eight times more common from 4:00 A.M. to 6:00 A.M. than during the day, even though there are three times as many trucks on the road during peak daytime hours.

In the week following the switch to Daylight Saving Time each spring, when people are forced to rise an hour earlier (and adjust their internal clock accordingly), there are 10 percent more traffic accidents than usual.

But the practice that is most difficult on the body is the rotating shift, as a study by Dr. Czeisler and several other sleep researchers has determined.

"Our findings have major implications for both industry and labor," reports Dr. Czeisler, who has developed the Center for Design of Industrial Schedules, a nonprofit organization. He said the study showed that employee turnover, illness, absenteeism, job safety and productivity are all significantly affected by rotating-shift work.

First of all, shift work in general affects employees adversely because it disturbs the biological clock, Dr. Czeisler says. But the study team found that workers adjust best to shift changes that move them to later starting times—morning shift followed by afternoon and night shifts instead of vice versa—because it more easily conforms to the biological clock. He says that workers are more efficient if their shifts are not rotated too frequently—three- or four-week shifts instead of one-week shifts.

The study began in 1981 after workers at the Great Salt Lake Minerals and Chemicals Corporation plant in Ogden, Utah, complained of insomnia, fatigue, digestive disorders and falling asleep on the job. The workers had been changing shifts every week, often to a shift that began earlier than the previous one.

The study group compared 85 male rotating-shift workers with a control group of 68 male nonrotating day- and swing-shift workers with comparable jobs. The rotating-shift workers were divided into two groups: 33 continued to change shifts every week, while 52 others were moved to a later shift every three weeks.

The research found that 81 percent of the 52 workers with the less frequent shift changes found they could adjust to altered sleep patterns in four days.

It appears also that less frequent shift changes make for a more satisfied employee. The nine-month study also determined that the rate of turnover among shift workers on

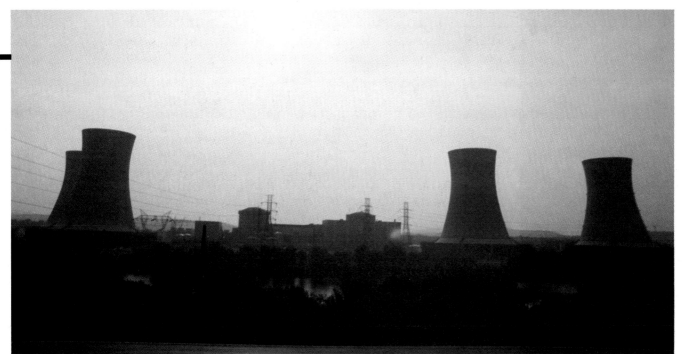

the three-week schedule dropped to almost the same level as that among those who did not change shifts. Fully 70 percent of the workers said they preferred the new system. In another study, conducted nationwide, Dr. Czeisler discovered that workers forced to change shifts at frequent intervals are often heavy users of sleeping pills, marijuana and alcohol as sleep aids. However, the use of such drugs can be expected to decline if shift changes conform more to natural body rhythms.

A PERIOD OF ADJUSTMENT

What can a worker on a weekly rotating shift do to avoid the energy drain of a disheveled schedule? Virtually nothing. "It takes about four days to adjust," says Dr. Czeisler. That's why a steady shift for three weeks is better than a one-week shift rotation. It allows the worker a time of normalcy.

Emphasizing that the body simply cannot make adjustments so abruptly without an energy drain, he noted further that "what you want to do in designing work schedules is to try to make it possible for the worker to adapt so he can be sleeping at a time when he can sleep most effectively and be functioning when he can be alert and awake."

Douglas K. Ayres, a research associate at the Center for Design of Industrial Schedules, reports that

subsequent studies have bolstered the conclusions reached in the Utah study.

"In measures of employee health, job satisfaction, accident rates, absenteeism and turnovers, the major principles developed have been very much borne out in practice," he said.

As to the most beneficial length of time between shift rotations, he said a change every three weeks was something of a compromise. "We actually came up with four weeks, but workers will not go to the ends of the earth in accepting the social limits of certain shifts. A three- or four-week schedule is most favorable both medically and socially."

Ayres also addressed another problem common to rotating-shift workers—gastrointestinal disorders. "Rotating-shift workers don't generally have regularly scheduled meals. They tend to eat alone more and tend to eat food of a lesser quality—junk food. Or, they might wake up at 8 o'clock at night and eat dinner with the family when the body expects breakfast."

And, he added, rotating-shift workers tend to exercise less because their energy level has been drained by their irregular hours.

Ideally, nobody should work rotating shifts. Realistically, that is impossible. The best compromise, then, is a shift schedule that keeps employees working as close to peak energy levels as possible.

The place: Middletown, Pennsylvania. The date: March 28, 1979. And the time was 4:00 A.M. —halfway through the midnight shift—when the crew at Three Mile Island got the first hint that the worst nuclear power plant accident in history was under way. Could the "error" have had anything to do with the erratic schedule of the shift workers? Quite possibly, says Charles Ehret, Ph.D., chronobiologist with the Argonne National Laboratory in Illinois. "The crew members had been on a schedule of weekly shift changes when the accident occurred," says Dr. Ehret. He and other scientists believe that rotating shifts such as the ones then in effect at TMI reduce the efficiency of workers.

TV News: A Rude Awakening

You say you're in the habit of jumping into bed each night at 11:00 and catching the late news and maybe a news talk show before dropping off to sleep? Well, that may or may not be a good idea. Watching late-night news programs can interfere with a good night's sleep if you find yourself getting too involved with them.

"If the show turns on your thought processes and you're the kind of person who finds it difficult to 'turn off' your mind afterward, then these programs could make it harder to fall asleep," reports June M. Fry, M.D., Ph.D., director of the sleep disorders center at the Medical College of Pennsylvania.

What's more, says Jerome L. Singer, Ph.D., a Yale University psychologist, "Yes, they can get into your dreams. So if your dreams are bad enough to wake you up, that's obviously not good for your sleep."

Thus, if you find yourself staring at the ceiling after turning off the 11 o'clock news, it might be better to wait until morning to find out what's happening in the world.

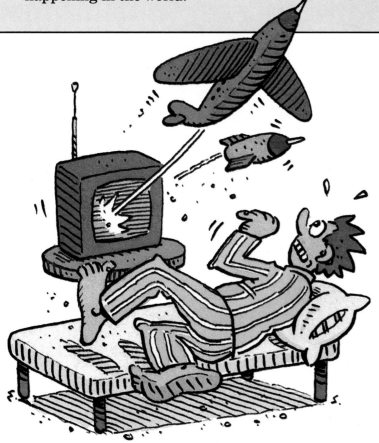

believe they are sleeping soundly at night.

Narcolepsy (literally, "numbness seizure") is a chronic sleep disorder that usually appears during adolescence and has no known cause or cure. It takes its name from its most common symptom, the irresistible desire to fall asleep, often at inappropriate moments—like when you're driving a car. It is frequently accompanied by a feeling of exhaustion.

According to American Narcolepsy Association president William Baird, "If every day it seems necessary to take a nap, and between naps you feel tired, dragged out and exhausted, narcolepsy might very well be the problem."

If you suspect you have a sleep disorder, it's best to consult your physician.

YOUR SLEEPING ENVIRONMENT

For some of us, however, it may not be a medical condition that disturbs our sleep. It may be our surroundings—like a lumpy bed or a street light glowing through the window or, heaven forbid, pink and orange giraffes romping all over the wallpaper. It could mean it's time for a change (or in extreme cases, an interior decorator).

Never underestimate the importance of your sleeping environment. Unfortunately, with the common necessity of at least occasional travel and the noise level of urban living, it's not always possible to create the absolute ideal in sleeping quarters.

But there are important steps each person can take. The idea, of course, is to make your bedroom a warm and inviting place where refreshing sleep comes easily and naturally. You can create this atmosphere with careful choice of room decoration and bed, and by ensuring that room temperature and bed clothes are suited to your personal needs.

The crucial point to remember in selecting a sleeping environment is that there is no one governing set of instructions. What is comfortable and relaxing for you might keep someone else tossing and turning all night long.

Some people feel most secure sleeping with a light on. Others like to create the darkest, quietest atmosphere possible. Some people sleep best with a pet or a partner; others require a solitary sleeping atmosphere. Windows open or windows closed? It's up to you as long as you don't create an environment so warm or so cold as to interfere with your sleep.

Generally, a quiet atmosphere is the best for restorative, uninterrupted sleep. If you live in an area that is unusually noisy at night, or if your schedule forces you to sleep during the daytime, you can help to insulate your atmosphere by putting heavy drapes on the windows.

While there are many important ingredients that go into the making of a good night's sleep, there is one that should never be ignored. That is the bed or, more specifically, the mattress. We tend to grow attached to our beds and perhaps fail to notice that the mattress is losing its resilience and beginning to sag. Yet improper support can lead to a whole host of annoyances that steal sleep and sap energy.

According to Robert G. Addison, M.D., clinical associate professor of orthopedic surgery at Northwestern University Medical School and director of the center for pain studies of the Rehabilitation Institute of Chicago, "All night long as you sleep on a too-soft or too-hard bed, your muscles are working overtime to align your spine. It's no coincidence that many people wake up in the morning with a backache. They haven't given those muscles any time off to rest."

Sleep is the largest period we go through in a prone position, says Lionel A. Walpin, M.D., clinical director of physical medicine and rehabilitation at Cedars-Sinai Medical Center in Los Angeles, and we have the least control over it. "We turn over rapidly dozens of times during the night and can stress tight muscles without even knowing it. Then, to make matters worse, we remain in contorted positions for long periods of time—putting additional strain on muscles, tendons, ligaments, nerves and joints."

Even though doctors recognize the problems the wrong bed can create, they can't agree on a single solution. That's because there isn't one—there are many.

"No bed is perfectly suited for everyone," notes Dr. Addison, who has helped design mattresses for major bedding firms. "However, the ideal mattress should cradle the spine in the same position as if you were standing with good posture."

In most cases, the key word in mattresses is firm. Body weight is not evenly distributed, so adequate support is needed for those parts that sink deepest into the mattress—hips, chest and head in particular. Not all mattresses are created equal, however, so not all of them distribute weight in the most desirable way.

While it is impossible to recommend a single bed and mattress that is best for everyone, there are some guidelines that can help people to a more comfortable night's rest.

Dr. Walpin believes that "versatility in all bedding products is the ideal." He has helped to develop a unique pillow that offers four different degrees of head and neck support simply by turning the pillow around and over.

Most important, a bed and mattress should not be bought in haste. This is a purchase that requires time and attention. "If you have to try out a mattress in the store," advises Dr. Addison, "lie down on it for 10 minutes at least. Study what happens to the bed as you vary your position. When you lie on your back, your buttocks should be supported and you should feel the support. You should be able to lie comfortably on your stomach without unnaturally arching your back, although I don't recommend this as a primary sleeping position. On your side, your shoulders and hips should sink in slightly so that your spine settles in a horizontal, not a curved, position."

While all of this careful checking may seem like a pain in the neck to the clerk in the store, it may avoid a permanent one for you in the long run.

In fact, all aspects of sleep and the sleeping environment should be taken seriously, for this precious commodity is one of nature's prime ways of assuring you a long, healthy and happy life.

Don't take your sleep lightly.

Pillow Talk

A quick primer on pillows: For best rest, back sleepers should use a thin, soft pillow. So, too, should side sleepers, unless they have broad shoulders. In this case, a thicker pillow is called for. The best pillow will discourage stomach sleeping, since that posture puts pressure on your jaw and irritates neck muscles.

Read This and Fall Asleep

This story has designs on you. It's neither tale nor treatise nor tract, but a kind of spell, a potion on paper that pulls you toward that realm that all insomniacs yearn for: sleep.

No, don't look for the secret to this sleight of hand, for looking can only keep you awake. Don't expect elaborate explanations of how the words reach into your brain's sleep center and flip the switch to "snooze." There won't be any. The following sentences are psychotechniques in motion, calibrated to the rules of autogenic training, self-hypnosis, systemic desensitization and progressive muscle relaxation. And that's all you need to know. Nothing else matters if you really want sleep to come.

So prepare yourself. Let your body—not the clock—whisper that it's bedtime. Take the phone off the hook, set the house thermostat to 64°F, soothe yourself in a hot bath, drink a glass of warm milk (just as you did when you were a child), dim the lights (you need barely enough light to read by), make that last trip to the bathroom and go to bed as you always do. Lie in a comfortable position and use a pillow to prop this book in front of you.

Now, just read, read as you would a novel or a poem, without looking for information or advice or an answer to anything. Your eyes descend on every word in slower and slower time; it matters little whether you ever get to the last sentence, for every line is a concluding remark.

Slower. Every period of each sentence you pass signals your mind to reduce your reading pace. And there's no place you have to be, no problems you have to solve now. Tomorrow will wait for tomorrow, and you'll meet it better after this good night's rest.

Just say yes. Ever so softly, whisper it now: yes. Say it when you're tempted to analyze what you're reading. Say it when you start to wonder if this spell will work. Say it and give up your last ounce of resistance to these words and the sleep lurking between the lines. Say it without trying to make anything happen, without expecting to doze off, without caring whether sleep comes or not. Just say it: yes.

And breathe deeper, letting your chest rise and fall slowly in even rhythm. Beneath the surface of these words should flow the currents of your breaths, long and sturdy, air easing in, air easing out. And if you listen to them long enough, you'll see how discrete each one is, each one with a slightly different depth or duration or strength. When you come to the end of this paragraph, close your eyes and listen to them until you start to distinguish one from another. It may take you 10 seconds or 10 minutes. And when you open your eyes, that slow current of respiration will seem steadier than before, and you'll hear it more as you continue reading, and it will flow on its way with the words that flow from left to right.

You're lying on the white sands of a beach that stretches to meet a clear sky. There is only sand the color of snow and sky the color of robins' eggs. Your eyes are closed, and you feel the rays of a sun that warms but does not burn and a breeze that brings along salty sea air.

Place your right arm at your side and clench your fist. Right now. Tense every muscle as hard as you can—your wrist, forearm, upper arm. Feel the tension build as the muscles strain and burn. Feel it. Now listen to your breathing in the background. Wait for one of those slow exhalations. Wait. Now let your arm go limp as you exhale. Feel the muscles loosen up, feel the heaviness, enjoy it. Your arm hasn't been this relaxed all day.

Now do the same thing with your left arm: Tense, hold the tension, then relax as you exhale. It feels so good you want to close your eyes to savor it. And you will close them, but not yet.

Tense your scalp, face, neck and shoulders. Tighten your scalp as if someone were giving your head a vigorous shampoo. Push your tongue against the roof of your mouth, wrinkle your nose, purse your lips, clench your back teeth. Freeze your neck muscles and thrust your shoulders toward your ears. Now you're holding your breath, and your taut muscles are just starting to ache. Hold the tension. Just a little longer. Now go limp and exhale. Let your mouth fall open, your head droop slightly as gravity wills. Feel the heaviness in the muscles, the spreading warmth. Listen to the slow, slow march of your breaths toward long rest.

As you lie on the long, white shore you hear only the muffled rasp of ocean waves far away, and from the sun that doesn't burn comes warm yellow light that bathes you, down to every cell. The rays melt tension and calm your thoughts.

Slowly arch your back as you take in a breath and hold it. Now stiffen your spine and push your chest forward, letting tension course through the muscles. Wait for a count of 5. Now release tension and exhale. Feel the wave of relaxation wash over your muscles as you let your breathing even out again. Your body has never seemed so heavy, so warm. You can hardly move. It takes great effort just to turn the page.

Think now of the muscles in your abdomen, your stomach, your buttocks, your hips. Wait for a languid exhalation. There. Stop breathing and squeeze the muscles in your stomach and abdomen, contract every sinew in your buttocks and hips, make your midsection harden to stone. Tense every fiber as hard as you can. Let the tension build. And build. Now release the strain and exhale. The muscles loosen and now you can't feel them, just the heaviness of stone, the warmth of ease, the slow rising and falling of your chest.

Listen for one of those inhalations. Listen. And hold it. Hold it and tense your legs and feet. Straighten your legs and bend your ankles, pointing your toes upward toward your knees. All these muscles are now as stiff and hard as wood. Keep them rigid. Now exhale and let them go limp, letting the tension seep away. Let them relax until they can't relax any further. Then relax them some more, and hear the muffled rasp of your steady breathing.

You feel warm all over, your whole body is lead, every muscle is now cousin to sleep. And yes, at the end of this paragraph you can close your eyes. And only if you open them again before morning should you keep reading these words that crawl from left to right.

The waves are rolling louder now, swelling in the yellow light, then splashing on the warming sands. You lie still, listening to the surf as it draws back, then washes in, like the sound of air easing out of your chest, then flowing in again.

There's something here that tranquilizes the brain, nudges it toward natural sleep. . . . Deepen your breathing, slowly pulling in all the air you can, gently pushing out all that's possible. There. Now do it again. And again: Take in a roomful of air, a houseful. . . . Now expel it, emptying out every trace of breath. Stop. Hold till your chest strains for air. Now release.

This gorging and clearing your lungs, then holding your breath, is the opiate for slumber, and when you come to the end of this paragraph, you'll indulge. You'll close your eyes and repeat the pattern until your body's desire for normal breathing overwhelms the long breaths. All the while you'll have your eyes turned upward, as though watching a scene at the back of your head. You'll imagine each of those grand breaths drawing in warm and yellow air, air that enters through your right foot, seeps up your leg into your chest and neck, down through your left leg and out your foot.

On the white sand you lie leaden, basking in the thick, yellow warmth, hearing the splash and roar of the talking sea. In rhythmic rounds of swaying water, it says something, something you can't quite make out . . .

Say it: *I'm a breath away from sleep.* Yes, whisper it now: *I'm a breath away from sleep.* Exhale: *sleep.* Exhale: *sleep.* Exhale: *sleep.* As the waves crest and fall on those white sands in your mind, think it. As you lie there in the drowsy warmth of the sand, as the scene curls up to a soft yellow glow, think it: *sleep.*

Sleeper's Q & A

Q Will activity at bedtime—like exercise or sex—help me sleep or keep me awake?

A It depends on the activity. While exercise during the day or early evening will help you sleep later on, it's generally believed that exercise right before bed has such a stimulating effect on the body that it makes the immediate onset of sleep difficult. But that rule does not necessarily apply to sex. The general rule concerning sex and sleep is this: Satisfying sex leads to satisfying sleep. Sex complicated by feelings of physical or emotional inadequacy can, however, contribute to insomnia.

Q Will I need to sleep *more* if I take up exercise?

A No. You may even find yourself needing to sleep less. "I've seen a lot of executive types take up exercise," reports Allan Ryan, M.D., editor-in-chief of *The Physician and Sports Medicine,* "and found that exercise, if anything, reduces the amount of time people need to spend in bed by helping them to fall asleep in the first place."

What happens is this: Exercise exhausts your muscles. And it's physical exhaustion that introduces you to stage one of the sleep cycle—a kind of semiconsciousness that leads to progressively deeper stages of sleep, culminating in the all-important dream state.

Q I hate to take sleeping pills but sometimes I feel I need something to help me fall asleep. Is there anything I can take that won't give me the hung-over feeling I sometimes get from the sleeping pills?

A Yes. Many researchers are now convinced that tryptophan has sedative properties that may be helpful to people with occasional sleep problems.

Tryptophan *(TRIP-ta-fan)* is one of the 20 amino acids contained in protein foods. After it enters your body through the food you eat, some of it turns into a brain compound called serotonin, which aids sleep. Does that mean a glass of warm milk (or any other protein food, for that matter) before bed really will help insomnia?

Well, not exactly. It's a little more complicated than that. You do get tryptophan from protein foods, but when you get it in that form, it's directly competing with eight other amino acids for access to the brain. The other amino acids defuse tryptophan's effect on serotonin levels, so it loses a lot of its knockout effect on sleep.

But you can take pure tryptophan—without the competing amino acids—in tablet form.

Ernest Hartmann, M.D., professor of psychiatry at Tufts University School of Medicine in Massachusetts and renowned sleep researcher, has spent years researching tryptophan and its effect on serotonin and sleep. In various experiments performed at the sleep laboratory and sleep disorders center he directs, Dr. Hartmann has now found that doses as low as 1 gram help mild insomniacs and people who have trouble falling asleep in strange places.

So here are Dr. Hartmann's suggestions for treating sleeplessness: Take 1 to 2 grams of tryptophan about 45 to 60 minutes before bed (tryptophan takes a little while to affect your serotonin levels). Don't be disappointed if you don't feel its effect on the first or second night. Many people don't see effects for two to three weeks after starting it. When it does take effect, you can cut your dosage to three to four days on, then three days off, says Dr. Hartmann. (Of course, this or any other supplement program should have your doctor's okay.)

Q Is it possible to make up lost sleep?

A Sure. It works like this. Suppose you've slept only 6 hours a night during the week, but you usually get 8 hours. By Friday, you'd be 8 hours short. But to make up for your lost sleep you don't have to sleep an extra 8 hours—or a grand total of 16 hours at a shot in the sack. Instead, your body cleverly rushes you through the light stages of sleep, cuts down a bit on dream time and gets you right to stage four—that's when you're "dead to the world." The percentage of total sleep time spent in stage four is increased. As a result, you achieve a restorative night's sleep—with just a little overtime on the pillow.

So, if you're planning a long weekend where fun and more fun—not rest and relaxation—is the primary goal, a good night's sleep at the end of it all should be enough to prepare you to face the world again Monday morning.

Q My sleeping problem is my husband, who repeatedly awakens me during the night with his snoring. Are there any snoring remedies?

A There are a lot of snoring remedies, but it's difficult to tell which one might work for your husband. Here are a few that doctors have found to be effective in some cases.

Prop up the head of your bed by putting a brick or two under the two legs. This elevates the snorer's head and helps keep the airway open. Don't use extra pillows—they'll only kink the airway.

Absolutely avoid using central nervous system depressants, such as alcohol, tranquilizers, sleeping pills or antihistamines, late in the day.

Lose weight and exercise regularly.

Wear a cervical collar, the kind that's prescribed for people with sprained necks. Most snoring occurs when the sleeper lies on his back with his chin resting on his chest. That narrows the windpipe. The collar keeps the chin up and the windpipe open.

Q I have found my young son walking in his sleep on several occasions, a habit which I had as a child and which I experience once in a great while to this day. Is this a sign of deeper problems? Can I do anything about it?

A It has been determined that sleepwalking runs in families, and that a tendency toward it is almost certainly inherited. It does not signify serious psychological problems any more than occasional nightmares do. However, it has been found that people tend to sleepwalk at times when there is tension in their waking life.

In adults, other causes of sleepwalking include alcohol intake before bed and the use of various drugs that act on the nervous system.

When scientists measured the brain waves of sleepwalkers, they found, not surprisingly, that they are only half asleep (or half awake, depending on how you want to look at it) and function like people with diminished capacities. Because of this, special precautions should be taken in homes where sleepwalkers live. If possible, the sleepwalkers should be allowed the use of first-floor bedrooms. Windows to which they have access should be made difficult to open. It's also helpful to remove sharp obstructions from the sleeping area because sleepwalkers have a tendency to bump into things.

We know of one case in which a family—disturbed by the nocturnal room-to-room wanderings of a teenage daughter—sealed the doorway of her room each night with newspaper. When the girl walked through the paper she woke herself up and merely went back to bed. The rest of the family was able to sleep in peace.

5

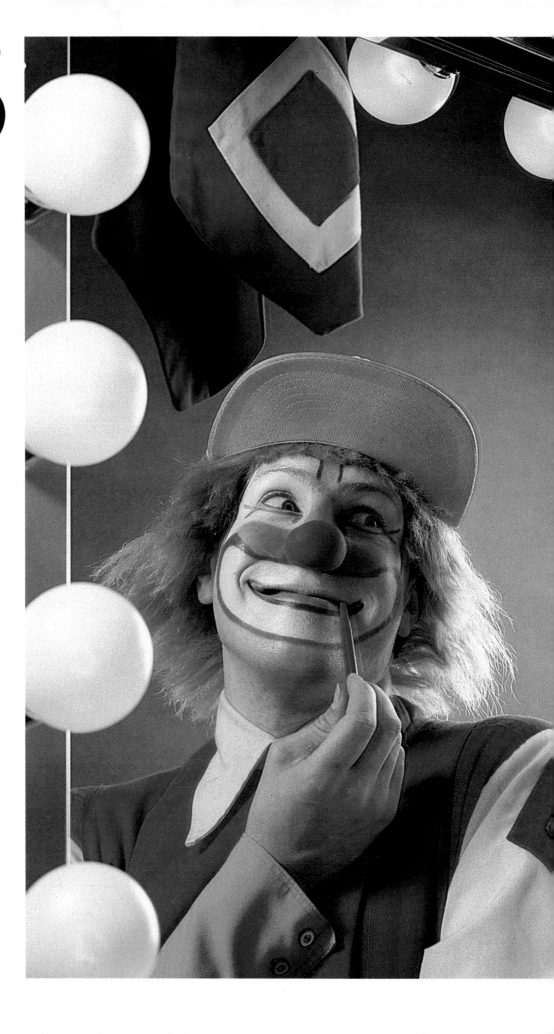

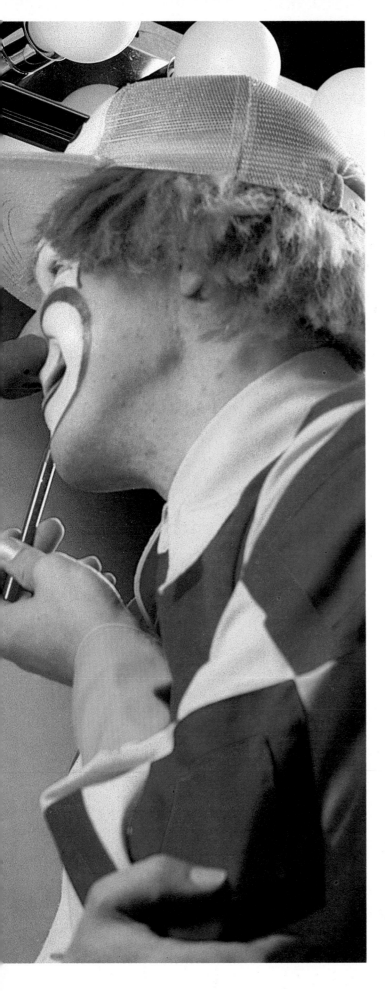

Attitude Makeovers

Take a good look at yourself from the inside out. You may find those elusive energy drainers are all in your head.

H ow does the bee fly? Scientists have been intrigued by that question for decades. Using formulas that work for birds and planes and other flying insects, scientists could "prove" on paper that the bee can't fly—not enough wing, too much body weight. Yet the bee, knowing nothing of science, flies.

What's intriguing about this story is this—if the bee could think, if it could be convinced by "experts" that it could not fly, would it try anyway?

If it were human, it might not. Unlike the bee, our species does think.

And unlike the bee—whose life is ruled by repetitive behavior patterns that have been imprinted on its genes over millions of years—we have to *choose*. Yet negative attitudes—feeling listless, uncreative, down on ourselves—can sap our energy so much that we can sit in front of a job we know we have to do, yet not be able to muster the desire to even begin.

How can we get back that high-energy buzz, that try-and-stop-me attitude? Well, if we want our lives to take off, we have to learn what's holding us down. We have to dissect the negative attitudes that keep our enthusiasm grounded. It's not a pretty picture, but don't worry. In a few pages, you're going to learn how to cover it with a fresh coat of paint.

THE POWER OF POSITIVE ACTION

Negative attitudes. Shakespeare's Hamlet is the worst-case scenario, the direct opposite of the busy bee, as he wallowed in his indecision, always finding the best reasons *not* to do anything about his lot in life, even though he felt himself the victim of great injustice. So caught up was he in feelings of helplessness that he spent most of his time agonizing over what to do and what not to do, and he never got around to doing anything.

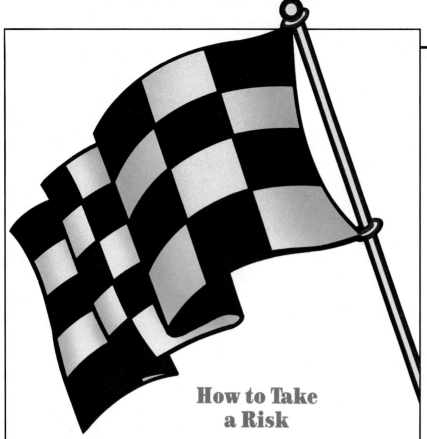

How to Take a Risk

"Not risking is the surest way of losing," says California psychiatrist David Viscott, M.D., author of *Risking*. "It eventually destroys your life. You never learn who you are, never test your potential, never stretch or reach. You become comfortable with fewer and fewer experiences."

Any risk, he says, can be thought of in three parts: preparing, committing and completing. To explain, he likened a calculated risk to passing another car on the highway, probably the most dangerous maneuver in driving.

First, you have to recognize your need to risk, and that's always threatening because you're forced to admit your present situation must change. Stuck behind an unpredictable or drunk driver, you may decide to pass because staying where you are is more dangerous than taking that risk.

Because the decision to risk means leaving something behind, "you've got to figure out what things you're going to lose and accept that, so it doesn't become a negative force later on."

Step two is putting your plan into action, committing to the risk. "Take your time getting ready, but when you go for it, don't let up until you're sure everything is in place," Dr. Viscott advises.

And finally, the third step, completion: You swing back into your own lane, exhilarated and a little shaken, mission accomplished.

Most of us find ourselves caught somewhere in between the busy bee buzzing about his business and Hamlet's "To be, or not to be."

We cope. We deal with what we have to in our daily lives. We steer the course of our own lives, more or less, and feel pretty good about it. But there are times—and everybody has them—when things seem to slip out of control. Life seems to be steering us instead of vice versa. We can call it job burnout or think of ourselves as living in a rut. But whatever we call it or whatever its cause, it's not pleasant. We feel uncomfortable, uneasy, bored, depressed, unsure of ourselves. And it can get worse.

It makes us worry about what's wrong with us—where did we lose it? The more we fret, the worse we feel, and the tougher it becomes to do anything about it. And it won't go away on its own.

"The result," says Gary Emery, Ph.D., director of the Los Angeles Center for Cognitive Therapy, "is a vicious cycle. You wind up doing things you don't like, and not doing things you do like, and your self-image, your sense of independence, suffers."

And if you thought you had problems before, now you've *really* got them. Your attitude is decidedly negative and your energy is running out. You hardly have the strength to face all that seems wrong with your life, and you start thinking in terms of excuses and blame. "It's not my fault I'm miserable—that husband/wife of mine never lets me up for air." Or, "Why should I even kid myself about my chances for promotion? I should have gotten my degree like my father wanted me to. Why didn't I listen to him? Why didn't he push me more?"

What to do? What to do? "If you wait around until you like yourself, you'll wait forever," says Dr. Emery, who is author of *A New Beginning: How You Can Change Your Life through Cognitive Therapy* and *Own Your Own Life: How the New Cognitive Therapy Can Make You Feel Wonderful.*

"Just doing something seems to be the most powerful thing," he says. And the first step is to change the way you *think.*

Cognitive therapy, which holds that we are what we think, "seeks to correct errors in thinking which contribute to a variety of personal problems," says Dr. Emery. If negative thoughts compound themselves in a downward spiral of indecision, self-doubts and loss of energy and will, then positive thoughts—and positive actions—can reinforce each other in an ascending spiral of energy and accomplishment.

NO IFS, ANDS OR BUTS

The first step toward a positive approach to life, says Dr. Emery, is to decide what you want out of your life, then to realize that it's your choice.

How to do that? The trick is being able to determine what the real obstacles are and to separate them from the ones your mind has worked up. And to do *that,* you have to get rid of the "what-ifs" and the "if-onlys." By using those phrases you are excusing yourself from having to make a decision on some pretty phony grounds. *What if* you do call that special someone and you do get put down? Ouch! But what if you never call? Really, is that going to make you feel any better about yourself? *If only* you had listened to your father and gone to college. Well, you *didn't*—but where is all this wishful thinking getting you? If only life were fair, nobody would get old and wrinkled, and we'd all be rich. Obviously, there is something awry about the "what-if, if-only" line of reasoning—it doesn't go anywhere because it doesn't have anything to do with reality.

Simply put, no blame, no excuses—no ifs, ands or buts. "Everybody has excuses, millions of them," says Dr. Emery. "You have to accept all of them for what they are, act like they don't exist, and go do it. If you don't, you've made a decision anyway. In deciding not to decide, you've decided not to go after what you want out of your life. The problem isn't going to go away, and if you're going to agonize that much over it, you owe it to yourself to reassess just what it is that you are doing to yourself."

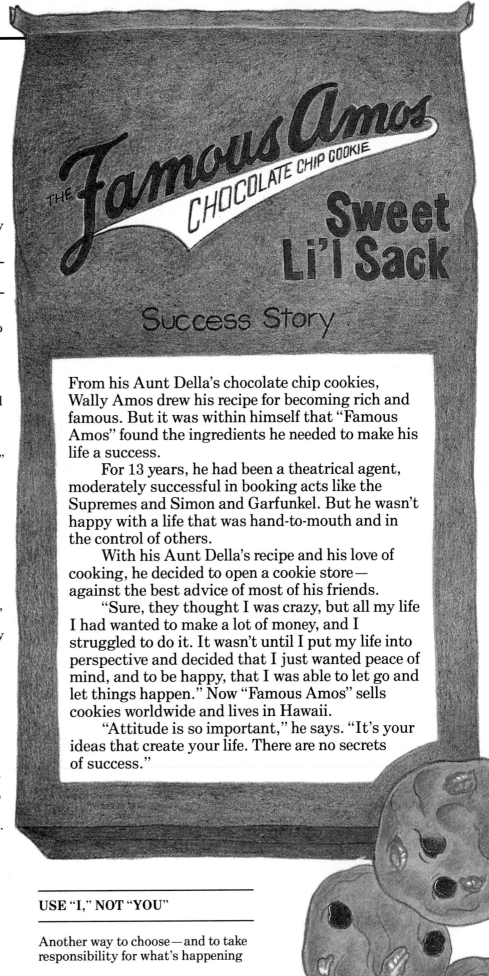

THE *Famous Amos* CHOCOLATE CHIP COOKIE

Sweet Li'l Sack

Success Story

From his Aunt Della's chocolate chip cookies, Wally Amos drew his recipe for becoming rich and famous. But it was within himself that "Famous Amos" found the ingredients he needed to make his life a success.

For 13 years, he had been a theatrical agent, moderately successful in booking acts like the Supremes and Simon and Garfunkel. But he wasn't happy with a life that was hand-to-mouth and in the control of others.

With his Aunt Della's recipe and his love of cooking, he decided to open a cookie store— against the best advice of most of his friends.

"Sure, they thought I was crazy, but all my life I had wanted to make a lot of money, and I struggled to do it. It wasn't until I put my life into perspective and decided that I just wanted peace of mind, and to be happy, that I was able to let go and let things happen." Now "Famous Amos" sells cookies worldwide and lives in Hawaii.

"Attitude is so important," he says. "It's your ideas that create your life. There are no secrets of success."

USE "I," NOT "YOU"

Another way to choose—and to take responsibility for what's happening to you—is to listen to how you talk, to the words you use to explain your feelings and frustrations: "You make me so mad because you're so insensitive. You just take me for granted."

Talking to someone with these "you" messages, especially when we express our frustrations and inner feelings, reveals a lot about the attitudes we use to face the difficult emotional situations and choices of our lives. It shows that we feel someone else controls us, that our emotions are puppets and someone else holds the strings. We feel passive, like a victim. In short, we *blame*. But there's another way.

If you want to take control of your own feelings in such situations, simply change the way you express yourself to more realistically define what is actually happening to *you*.

Instead of, "You make me so mad," try this: "I am angry because you spent your entire time at the party last night talking to the guys/girls about sports/gossip, and I become upset when you pay no attention to me every time you get close to your friends."

Big difference. In the last example, there's no blaming. You are simply discussing the specifics of a situation you don't like. Not only are you claiming control of your own feelings and your own life, you're also laying the groundwork for a much more productive discussion. Such an approach provides an opportunity to avoid a bitter argument that does nothing but rehash a past history of slights and put-downs and leaves you exhausted and feeling bad about yourself. And it frees your partner from feeling defensive and blaming you in turn. Instead, your partner can talk about his or her feelings. It's two adults choosing to share instead of two children striking out.

THE SECRETS OF SUCCESS

Ambition—just what is it we want to make of our lives? For many of us, that's the toughest "attitude" question of all. Perhaps we know we're not where we want to be. Or we know we're not doing what we want to day by day. But in an age that offers so much in the way of choice, it's not easy to decide which of the opportunities life presents to us is for us.

Not knowing which direction to take can be just as debilitating as any other of our self-doubts, draining our will, purpose and energy.

Some people, says Frederic F. Flach, M.D., a psychiatrist at Cornell University Medical College in New York City, may be where they want to be—yet *still* not feel satisfied. "Even though they have very good lives," he says, "some people find it very difficult to enjoy life."

Guilt, he explains, is one reason. "They feel they didn't earn it, or don't deserve it." Another reason is dissatisfaction—not with what we have but with what we don't have.

"We are truly victims of a marketing society," Dr. Flach explains. "We want things we don't need. Our society thrives on our discomfort."

In either case, Dr. Flach says, people have two choices—"They can either change their lifestyles or they have to change how they experience their lives and the way they view their own personal values."

In other words, learn to live with the good things life has given you, without guilt and without the dissatisfaction that often comes from knowing others have more. Or change the way you live to reflect what's in your mind—get a better-paying job, for instance, if you feel you can't afford everything you want. Or deal with your guilt in some way, perhaps by participating in projects that involve giving to others.

"Obviously," says Dr. Flach, "it's a lot easier to come to accept ourselves and our lives for what they are than to radically change them. Most people should be able to deal with their notions of guilt by realizing that some people will always be more fortunate than they are, and some always will be less fortunate. And most people should be able to realize the difference between what they really need in life and what they merely want. The purpose of advertising is to create the perception that our life is not complete without their product, but nobody needs a video recorder or a fancy sports car to survive or even to live quite nicely."

A Guide to Goal-Setting

Setting a course for life is much like sailing a boat on the open seas. A sense of direction is vital to avoid an aimless drift. Just as the sailor picks a destination and uses a compass and the stars to guide him there, we, too, need to set a direction for our lives and determine ways to measure our progress. We can do that by setting goals, both long term and short term.

"Goals give you direction and clarity," says cognitive therapist Gary Emery, Ph.D. "State the goal you want, and let it pull you. Making the big choices helps you make the little choices you have to make along the way," he explains.

Most people have little trouble setting their long-term goals—they want to be rich or famous, a lawyer or a doctor, a race car driver or a deep-sea diver. The problem comes from trying to figure out how to get from here to there.

Obviously, if you've never been to college and you want to be a brain surgeon or you don't have a driver's license and you want to be the winner of the Indianapolis 500, you've got your work cut out for you. The obstacles between you and your goal may seem insurmountable. And if you try to hurdle them all at once, they probably are.

But you don't have to do it all at once, advises Dr. Emery. If you break down your long-term goals into lots of short-term goals, each leading in the direction you want to go, you'll wind up facing not one enormous, insurmountable obstacle but a number of small, easily taken steps.

For example, say you want to be a lawyer but no 4-year college will consider your application for a prelaw course. What then? "You've got to keep your eye on your main goals and remain flexible," says Dr. Emery. "There are a million different ways to get where you want, so don't get discouraged if something you've been counting on doesn't work. Try something else." A 4-year college won't take you? Try a 2-year junior college to build up your academic credentials.

But what if you fail; what if you don't make it? Should you consider your life a failure because you fell short of your goal? If you end up with an associate degree instead of a law degree, you're still better off than if you had never tried. "You have to remember," says Dr. Emery, "that any job worth doing is worth doing poorly rather than not at all. Just doing what you can is better than doing nothing."

Below are some samples of one person's short- and long-term goals.

Short-Term Goals

1. I'm going to take a course in effective communications to help me get ahead at work.
2. I'm going to put myself on a realistic monthly budget so I can live within my means.
3. The next time there's a staff meeting, I intend to bring up that labor-saving idea I've been kicking around in my mind.
4. I'm going to improve my diet—get up earlier so I can fix myself a good breakfast, and I'm going to fix myself a salad for lunch instead of going out for pizza.

Long-Term Goals

1. I intend to go to law school some day, and a course in effective communications helps toward that goal.
2. My long-term goal is financial independence, so the obvious way to start is with a monthly budget.
3. There's no reason why I can't have a better job some day, but I'm going to have to demonstrate my leadership skills to get it.
4. I want to get back to what I weighed when I graduated from high school, and I want to do it before my next class reunion.

Don't Handcuff Your Creativity

"Just the facts, ma'am, just the facts." That's the way Sgt. Joe Friday approached the weekly crime riddles on television's "Dragnet."

While Sgt. Friday's analytical approach is a common method of problem-solving, experts say it's not the only way or even the best way. That's because this approach fails to tap the creative energies of the mind. It rules out new ideas because they've never been tried before and therefore there is no "factual" basis for analyzing them.

"Nobody knows what's possible until somebody tries something never tried before," says Gary Emery, Ph.D., a cognitive therapist. "If none of us had ever been willing to try our hunches and take a chance on the unknown, we'd all still be living in caves!"

So there's no need to apologize for your wild and crazy ideas—it's your creative energy at work!

DECIDING ON YOUR GOALS

For many of us, the problems we face are not a matter of guilt or dissatisfaction over our material possessions. Rather, they stem from living a day-to-day existence that seems to be going nowhere but into a rut—a dead-end job with no future prospects and no daily satisfaction, personal relationships that are unrewarding and unfulfilling, days spent listless, bored and pooped.

What we need in such a case is something to focus on, a goal that intrigues us and invites us to get our act together and our drive-train in gear. An ambition.

But where to find it? Life presents so many complex choices, from beekeeping to bookkeeping, and each one presents so many demanding requirements for success that it is vital that we understand where our talents and interests lie.

One good place to start is with recollections of our childhood, says Dr. Flach. "Everybody has a talent, and to find it, we have to look back. What games did you like as a child? What did you like in school?

"We pursue our talents spontaneously as children," he explains. "We tend to focus our energies on what we like to do, and what we like to do, we generally do well.

"But sometimes when we grow older, we make bad career choices, and the worse they are, the more trouble they get us into over the years."

In looking back to our childhood, we may discover that we exercised several talents and, even though we may have focused on one of them for a career choice, we may be able to bring others into play to expand our careers into areas which are much more rewarding.

In his own case, Dr. Flach notes that when he was a child, he found great satisfaction in writing—he published a small, neighborhood newspaper when he was in junior high school—and in the social service projects he became involved in through school programs.

"What I do as an adult," explains the psychiatrist/author, "is what I liked to do as a child. To me, doing both is much more satisfying than spending my time on either one alone, and as a result, both parts of my career have benefited."

ARE YOU DAYDREAMING?

But the past alone does not hold the key to unlocking our ambitions. The future constantly beckons, and most of us do spend time daydreaming about it, fantasizing about lifestyles and activities far removed from the daily grind.

But daydreams can provide us with more than just satisfying fantasies, says Dr. Emery. Daydreams can provide the clues to what it is we'd really like to be doing with our lives, he says.

"We can get a mental picture of where we'd like to be, and work from there," he explains.

Those mental pictures can come in different forms. Some show us a lifestyle we'd like for ourselves. Maybe we see ourselves driving a fancy sports car and wearing expensive clothes and jewelry. "If that's where we see ourselves at some point in our lives, then maybe it isn't a good idea for us to be thinking about spending our lives teaching or helping our fellow man, because we'll never make the kind of money we'll need to fulfill those inner needs," Dr. Emery explains.

And the opposite is just as true—if we daydream about saving the world from sickness or poverty, perhaps it's not a good idea to focus our careers on the business world and profits and losses, he says.

People also daydream about the kinds of activities they'd rather be doing—perhaps it's working in a woodshop, or flying an airplane, or arguing a case before the Supreme Court. No matter what the fantasy, there may be clues in our daydreams that are trying to tell us that the way we are spending our days is not the way we really want to, and that we might be happier, more ambitious and more energetic if we made a change.

And, Dr. Emery notes, it's never too late. "To get out of the rut, you have to realize that every moment is a fresh moment, a new start, and the past is the past."

The Creative Scenario

You don't have to paint murals to be creative, nor do you have to master the piano. Creativity should be a big part of your daily life, a major component in the way you tackle each day.

The truth is, *everyone* can be creative, say the experts. Creativity is finding new ways to approach old tasks and finding new uses for familiar items. You can start by telling yourself that there is no one correct way to do anything—even washing the dishes. Let your mind roam free to devise any number of different, interesting ways to handle even the most mundane chores.

Creativity can also help you handle problem situations. Below are a few examples with some typical and not-so-typical solutions.

Situation	Noncreative Solution	Creative Solution
It's raining cats and dogs and you've got to get to work. But you left your umbrella there yesterday.	Face up to getting to work soaking wet, or call the boss with your excuses.	Poke holes for eyes, nose and mouth in a plastic trash bag and wear it as a coat.
While changing a tire, you inadvertently kick all the lug nuts into a nearby storm sewer.	Spend 30 minutes trying to pry open the catch-basin before walking to the nearest phone.	Take one nut off each of the other three wheels and drive to the nearest garage.
The weather lifts in Chicago and lines are so long for the flight to New York it could take all day to board.	Complain to management, telling them you've just got to get to New York by dinnertime.	Take the first flight to Washington (no line), catch a shuttle and enjoy dinner in New York.
The kids drive you crazy all summer coming into the kitchen for drinks of water.	Give them plastic cups to use at outside faucets; clean up the litter.	Turn the outdoor faucet into a water fountain by reinstalling it upside-down.
It's a big night out, but both pairs of panty hose have an ugly run in one leg.	Make a mad dash to the drugstore, change in the car and arrive late, with a run in the new pair.	Snip the leg with the run from each pair. Wear both, turning one inside-out to match, if necessary.
While blowing bubbles, your child spills the container, then starts wailing.	Yell at the child, rush off for new container to stop the wailing.	Replace bubble solution with dishwashing liquid. Comfort child.
Your child's playball gets caught on a second-story roof.	Look for a ladder, swallow hard and start climbing.	Use a garden hose to "squirt" the ball off the roof.

67

FIND YOUR CREATIVITY

Daydreams, and the dreams we dream in the deep dark of the night, have long been thought to possess almost magical powers to restore the mind and soul, to provide almost mystical insights into the mysteries of life and to leave us refreshed and brimming with energy and purpose.

Dreams hold such magic for us because they well up from a side of our personalities that is instinctive, intuitive, highly visual and sensual and, above all, creative.

It also is a side of our personalities we rely on the least. Scientists know that there are two halves to the brain—two hemispheres. The left one controls the analytical, calculating side of our personalities. It is the storage house for the facts and figures of our lives—our language skills,

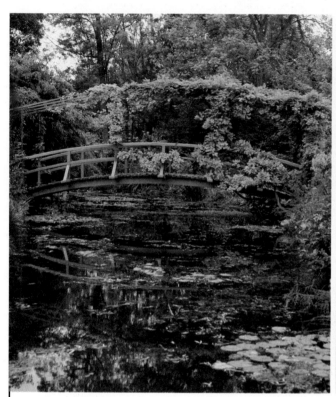 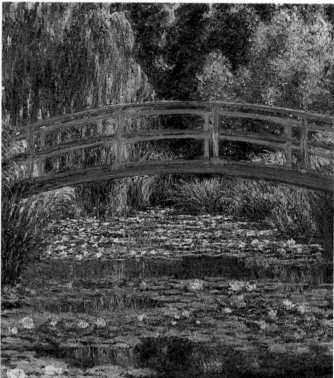

Your Creative Paradise

The best environment for putting out your best effort means different things to different people. French Impressionist painter Claude Monet, for example, found his inspiration in his garden at Giverny, shown in the photo at left above, which also became the scene of his famous painting *The Japanese Footbridge and the Water Lily Pond— Giverny,* shown at right above.

A creative environment can be anywhere, whether it's the company boardroom or your own backyard. It's what makes *you* feel good, it's where you feel comfortable, notes Frederic Flach,

M.D., a psychiatrist at Cornell University Medical College in New York City.

In looking for your creative environment, the important thing to remember is that the search itself should be no barrier to your creative efforts themselves.

"A lot of people complain they just can't be creative because they can't find the right atmosphere," says Dr. Flach, "but that's just a cop-out."

He also reminds us that creativity flourishes in a group environment. Brainstorming sessions to solve problems at work and group compositions in music are two prime examples.

grammar, vocabulary, multiplication tables and logic and reason. The right hemisphere of the brain operates in a much different manner—it is capable of transporting us to places we've never seen, places that have never been visited before by anyone. It is capable of playing an entire symphony in our minds, one that has never been played before by anyone. It tells us stories never before told and paints pictures never before seen. But most of us don't pay it much mind.

"We are a society of left-brain people," Dr. Flach explains. As children grow older, he explains, they are discouraged from "making things up." In school, the "right" answer is the only one that counts, and students are discouraged from taking individualistic approaches to mathematics, or science, or even art and literature. When students draw trees, for instance, they are expected to be green and brown, certainly not pink and purple, and, most of all, they are expected to look like trees. If a student deviates much from this norm, we begin to wonder if his different vision represents a learning disorder or some perceptual difficulty.

Yet the visions of the mind's eye are an essential part of a well-rounded life and an important tool to use in dealing with our day-to-day concerns, as well as the major problems everyone faces in life.

"It's an inherent part of the learning process for problem-solving and meeting life's challenges," says Dr. Flach. Though many people think of creativity in terms of artists and poets, Dr. Flach says that is not so. "We can be creative without possessing any particular artistic talent," he explains. A housewife, a plumber, an accountant—in fact, everybody— can benefit from innovative approaches to their work and their life, Dr. Flach says.

"Creativity can be applied in everyday life," according to the doctor. "When a child ties a shoelace for the first time, it's a creative act for him because he's never done it before. Creativity is the ability to put ideas together in new ways, to exchange one vision for a new and better one."

"Just about everyone," says Dr. Emery, "is creative in some area. It could be cooking dinner, taking care of kids, teaching." As Dr. Flach says, creativity is a matter of taking old ideas and putting them together in a new way. But Dr. Emery has a simpler, bolder instruction—"Make it up!"

"Everybody," he says, "wonders how Einstein, or Shakespeare, did it. And people study their lives, and the lives of other creative people, trying to find their secrets. But you can't look at creative people as experts on creativity because there's no one way. Why them and not others? Nobody knows.

"The truth is that there was nothing there when they began. They started out with nothing," Dr. Emery explains, "and they made it up as they went along."

It's a simple formula, Dr. Emery admits, but it can be extremely effective. "I know an author who, every time he plans on starting a new book, holds a dinner party to announce the title. He doesn't know what the book's going to be about—only that he's going to write one—and right out of the blue, he picks a title and announces it to his guests. He just makes it up, on the spot, but it provides the kind of motivation he needs to get his creative juices flowing to begin the project."

Though creativity is an obvious way to enhance the quality of our lives, Dr. Flach states that it is much more than that. Creativity, he says, is an essential ingredient to a complete, well-rounded personality. "I paint, I draw, I take photographs— not that I have any talent—because it exercises the right side of my brain, the visual or artistic side."

His goal is no different from anyone else's—creativity. He says it is crucial to developing a spontaneous personality.

Spontaneous. That's the word he uses to describe someone "who doesn't have to lie, even to himself, because he can face reality. He can tell the truth. He has a naturalness which comes from being comfortable with who he is."

That's the way most of us would like to see ourselves—assured, assertive, confident, motivated, ambitious and creative.

And, most of all, energetic.

Be Creative —It's Fun and Games!

Want to sharpen your creativity in a way that offers challenge, adventure and fun? Disregard the instructions, suggests Gary Emery, Ph.D. That's right. The next time you bring something home that has to be assembled—a child's toy, a wine rack, a wall unit— hide the instructions that come inside the box and try to wing it!

Sure, some of these things come with hundreds of pieces, scores of tiny little nuts and bolts and pages of instructions that are difficult at best. But as you lay out all the parts and envision just what it is these things are supposed to do when they're all assembled, you're putting the visual, creative part of your personality through a very vigorous and intriguing exercise.

Test Your Inner Strength

QUIZ

Do you have your act together? Assured? Assertive? Motivated? Ambitious? Creative? Not sure? Well, here's a quick and easy opportunity to take a measure of your inner strengths. There are no sneaky questions, so be honest with yourself—how would you react under similar circumstances?

1 The parking meter takes only quarters, but you have only dimes. So you:

    a. shrug your shoulders and walk off, figuring that if you get a ticket, it is, after all, a civic contribution

    b. buy cough drops at the drugstore even though you don't have a cough, so you can use the change to feed the meter

    c. ask the druggist for change for a dollar so you can feed the meter

2 Your boss takes you to his favorite fancy restaurant for lunch. The soup is too hot, the quiche is too cool, and the salad is limp. So you:

    a. bite your blistered tongue, smile bravely at the haughty waiter and tell your boss you can't wait to get back here with your spouse

    b. wonder aloud if you're going to need first aid for the blisters on your tongue, call the waiter "Buster" to let him know you didn't like the service and crank up the sarcasm to tell your boss that the lunch was an interesting experience if nothing else

    c. quietly tell the waiter the soup's too hot, the quiche too cool, and the salad limp, and that you'd like your lunch properly served

3 Your best friend asks if you wouldn't mind dog-sitting while she spends her 3-week vacation in Hawaii. She describes the beast as playful but you know he's really a holy terror and barely housebroken. You don't want to hurt her feelings. So you:

    a. tell her, "I'd love to," knowing full well that after 3 weeks of cleaning up after the destructive mutt you'll never want to speak to her again

    b. let her have it—ask her what makes her think that you're such a sap that you'd put up with that monster of hers for even a minute while she's off having a high old time in Hawaii

    c. tell her gently but firmly that you couldn't keep her pet because you don't have the time or the space to care for it the way she'd like

4 When you dream about the future, you see sandy beaches where in reality there is a laundry room piled high with dirty diapers, and a bright red sports car where there is really a broken-down station wagon with a hole in the muffler. You know your ambitions are far removed from your current reality. So you:

    a. dream on, spending a lot of time at the romance novel section of the local supermarket

    b. persuade yourself that your life isn't so bad and will get better some day, and tell yourself that sandy beaches and red sports cars are out of reach for most people anyway, unless they're born rich or are movie stars

    c. enroll in continuing education courses and spend a lot of time looking in the want ads for an opportunity to better yourself. You keep in mind that the guy who owns your company—along with a villa in the Bahamas—likes telling everyone he's a self-made man

See, no sneaky questions. You've probably got a pretty good idea of where you stand already.

If you got stuck on the *(a)* answers, you've got problems facing up to the fact that it's your life, and it's up to you to get the most out of it. Maybe you see yourself as the self-sacrificing sort, but you're not getting much out of it.

If you found yourself favoring the *(b)* answers, you recognize your rights, but you're not so sure about getting them. You haven't fully taken charge of your life. You tend to look for sure bets, or to blame what's wrong with your life on things outside of yourself.

If the *(c)* answers best describe you, congratulations. You have your act together. And if you picked all the *(c)* answers, consider yourself one in a million—most of us, if we're honest with ourselves, have to own up to some *(a)* or *(b)* answers.

5 The notice on the bulletin board says the company will pay for continuing education courses for any employee who wants to take them. The people you work with say it's a waste of time because no college can teach you the job. You want to get ahead, but you're not sure college is the answer. So you:

a. think it over and come to the conclusion that it would be a waste of time—there's no way you can ever catch up to the ones who already have their degrees

b. enroll, figuring it can't hurt and maybe it will impress your boss. But you drop out when you realize just how much time it takes out of your life

c. enroll and decide to stick with it, even though it means no more bowling on Tuesday nights and you're not quite sure where it's going to take you

6 When you face a problem that has to be solved, you confront such a bewildering array of advice from your friends that reaching the right decision seems almost impossible. So you:

a. present all the facts to someone you trust as an expert on the problem you're dealing with, and let yourself be guided by her advice

b. make a list of possible solutions, carefully eliminating all the wild and crazy ideas that have crossed your mind—you want to be sensible about this and not waste your time on frivolous thoughts that run contrary to your experience and to the expert advice you've gotten

c. trust your instincts, sleep on your intuition and arrive at a solution you feel will work for you, even if it is different. Analyze the reasons why you think it will work, and keep faith with it even when your friends say you're crazy

7 You've got a good job with steady work and long-term security. But it's a bore, going nowhere. A self-employed friend makes you an exciting offer in an area you've always had your eye on. But it means giving up your security and starting over again. So you:

a. tell your friend you'd love to, but can't—it wouldn't be fair to your family to risk their security on a new career

b. agonize over your indecision, bitterly letting your family know that if it wasn't for your responsibilities to them, nothing would hold you back—then say no

c. take the chance, but only after rationally discussing the risks versus the benefits with your friend and your family and letting everyone know that no matter what happens, you can always put the experience to good use in getting another good job

8 The springs are coming out of the sofa, the rug is worn through, and the cat has climbed the drapes once too often. So you:

a. buy a living room set like the one you've always admired at your sister's, a rug that reminds you of your mother's and drapes on sale at a discount store. Nothing quite goes together, but everyone's going to watch television anyway, right?

b. want to do everything in the best of taste, so you hang the expense and hire an interior decorator, then ban the family from ever setting foot in the room to preserve the expensive splendor for expected compliments from unexpected guests

c. stand in the middle of the room, visualizing what you'd really like it to look like. You shop to find the right pieces, carefully mixing and matching the things you'd like to see in the room. You have the cat declawed

6

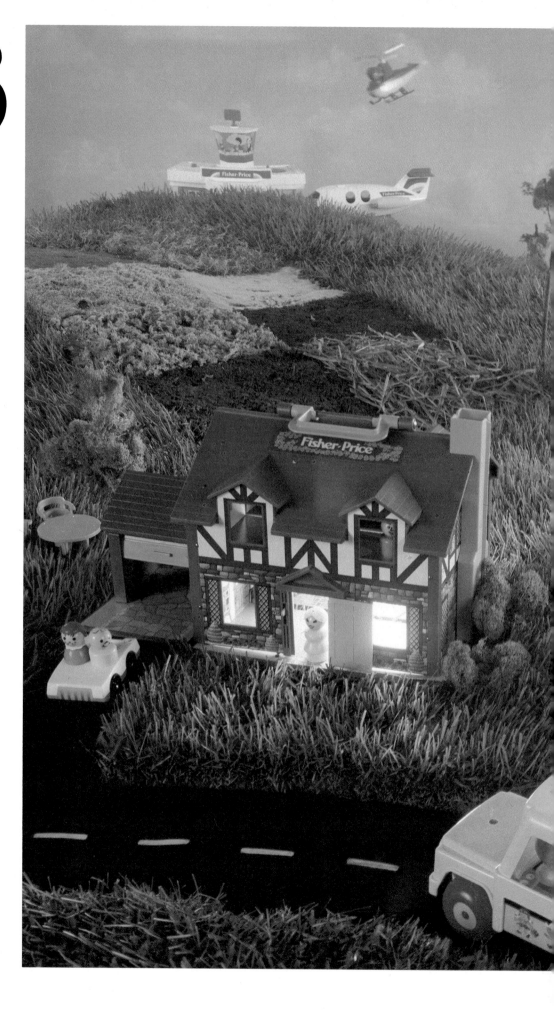

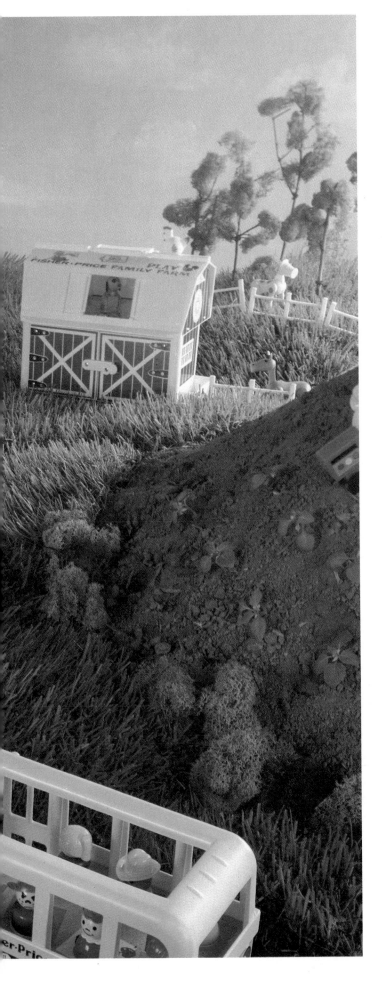

Extra-Energy Lifestyles

Living life to the limit depends as much on your resolve as your reserves. Learn how to keep low energy from putting your body on hold.

You seem to be doing everything right. A diet that makes your momma proud. A weight that makes your insurance agent smile. You exercise regularly. "I should be bounding with energy," you say, "but my basset hound has more vitality than I do! What gives?" It could be your lifestyle.

How's the marriage? Exciting as ever or flickering out? A fraying relationship can take the spring out of anyone's step. Marital advice is often controversial and highly charged. In fact, a charge might be exactly what you need.

And speaking of charges, how are things in the bedroom? Are they still honeymoon hot, or have they chilled to a Rodney Dangerfield level where you have sex the same way you have your steaks—rare? Maybe you're going about it all wrong.

Are the kids driving you nuts? Children gobble your energy like a famished horde of Pac Men sprung from their grids. Your attitudes toward child-rearing and your lofty expectations of life might be making you overreact, inviting their relentless attacks.

Is peering at the tube one of your escapes? Some respite. The free entertainment beamed magically into your home takes as much as it gives, and what it takes is your energy. You may be shocked to learn how much it strains and drains you and your kids.

Could it be a vacation that you need? Maybe. But be forewarned. Vacations can be relaxing, refreshing and reenergizing. They can also be frantic and frightfully fatiguing, and leave you even more frazzled.

Maybe for you, life just doesn't have the same spark since they pinned the final medal on your chest and pushed you out the door. The endless summer of retirement has dissolved into endless boredom, depression, lack of purpose and lost vitality. Cheer up. You've just fallen into a self-deprecation trap so common it's a cliche. In fact, it's tired old cliches about what you can and can't do anymore that are pounding your pep. Get out of that rocker and start living again.

A high-energy lifestyle will revitalize your happiness as well as your health. It can expand your horizons, unearth slumbering creativity and focus a fuzzy existence. It's your life. Live it to the limit? We'll tell you how.

MELANCHOLY MARRIAGES

Take my wife—please!
How's the wife? Compared to what?

A million jokes have been told since these two classics were first uttered, yet they remain as fresh and funny as ever. That's because the social problems they lambast, marital fatigue and boredom, remain as real today as in Henny Youngman's heyday. Probably even more so. With women taking their proper place in society, Joan Rivers is more than getting even with her hilarious "Take my husband—please" twists on the old theme.

The problem is, doctors, psychiatrists and sociologists aren't laughing quite so hard. A worn-out marriage can be both physically and emotionally devastating.

If cliches are your thing, doctors suggest tossing out "opposites attract" and holding to "birds of a feather," when it comes to marriage. In fact, abiding by the first adage may be fatal. A recent study concluded that Type A men—aggressive, impatient, active—have a greater risk of heart attack when married to Type B women—placid, cool, unruffled. The researchers found that it "may be psychologically and physiologically taxing for a husband who is hard-driving, competitive and ambitious to live with a woman who is the opposite."

Thyroid pioneer Broda Barnes, M.D., discovered that slow, listless hypothyroid victims were often drawn together in marriage. When one per-

son was cured, the marriage would be severely strained unless the partner was equally reenergized.

Psychiatrist Thaddeus Kostrubala, M.D., found similar problems developing between couples who differed in their levels of fitness. He said a strong element of jealousy and resentment can develop between fit/unfit couples. He suggests gently inviting the unfit partner to join in the fitness revolution, and then doing it together!

THE DUAL-CAREER DUEL

Another area of marital fatigue is the two-career couple. A quick rundown of factors that fatigue two-career marriages may help.

- A University of Minnesota study showed that the higher the disparity in a couple's income, the greater the chance of marital strain. Surprisingly, it didn't matter who had the higher salary, the husband or the wife. And in stark contrast to your mother's "marry a doctor" advice, the study says if a man or woman has two suitors, he or she should choose the one with a salary closer to their own.

- A study at Florida State University discovered that men vocally support sharing the housework with their working wives—that is, as long as they don't actually have to do it. (However, the study also pointed out that some women don't want their husbands to share the work.) While the media tell us that men have changed, the Florida study says women are not only bringing home the bacon, but cooking it, serving it and washing the pan. The study suggests that men should do less yapping and more scrubbing.

- Both partners in a dual-career marriage should have "enormous reserves of energy to be able to handle schedules that are frequently overloaded," advise Barrie S. Greiff, M.D., and Preston K. Munter, M.D., in their book *Tradeoffs*.

- "More fights in marriage are

over the issue of money (particularly the lack of it) than over any other issue," says time management expert Donna N. Douglass in her book *Choice and Compromise: A Women's Guide to Balancing Family and Career.* "More money is a possible advantage to a two-career marriage."

QUOTES, NOTES, ANTIDOTES

From the reams of self-help books and articles on marriage, we've gathered this selection of sage advice for keeping the energy up and the trouble down.

"There is good reason to believe that a later, more mature form of anything is better than its early, immature form. Love within marriage enjoys this process of ripening . . . ," writes Dr. Allan Fromme in *The Ability to Love.*

"Communication . . . is a very prevalent problem today. Many married couples live a sort of parallel relationship—side by side, rather than actually interacting. Resentments inevitably build up because they are never expressed. The result is . . . less intimacy," says Stanford R. Gamm, M.D., psychiatrist.

" 'When's dinner?' 'I'm hungry.' 'I don't have any clean socks.' These are service messages. This is not what a woman thinks of as communicating," says Dr. Joyce Brothers.

"Being honest and expressing all of your feelings is not always wise. The messages can be highly destructive— like 'your body disgusts me' or 'I'm in love with someone else,' " according to Carlfred Broderick, Ph.D., of the University of Southern California Human Relations Center.

"Nutrition is involved in 90 percent of my cases, and in 75 percent of them it's a major factor." Many marital spats, it seems, stem from hypoglycemia (low blood sugar), and sugar, refined flour and coffee are major culprits, says Mary Jane Hungerford, Ph.D., former director of the American Institute on Family Relations, Santa Barbara, California.

If all of these snares and potential troubles have you saying, "Why bother?" consider some of these statistics that have been collected over the years.

"The death rates from major diseases . . . are anywhere from two to six times higher for divorced men than married men. As compared to married women, widowed women have a 50 percent greater chance of dying from heart disease or stroke, twice the risk of dying from cancer of the cervix and four times the risk of dying in an auto accident," writes James J. Lynch, Ph.D., in *The Broken Heart: The Medical Consequences of Loneliness.*

Bachelors are admitted to mental hospitals 23 times more fre-

A Second Mate Can Rejuvenate the Golden Years

It's a familiar scenario—maybe even yours. The one-man woman or one-woman man is suddenly alone after death or divorce separates them from their long-time mate. "I'm too old, too tired to start again," they sigh. "Besides, Sid/Irma was the only one for me."

It's noble, but that kind of thinking can lead to a long, listless life, says a top gerontologist.

"One of the problems of getting older is the potential of ending up alone," says Holger Stub, Ph.D., a specialist in social gerontology from Temple University. "These people should strongly consider the revitalizing effects of remarrying."

You don't have to stay in a bad marriage just because it's lasted 30 years. "People hang on to bad marriages in their later years for many reasons, most of them wrong," says Dr. Stub. "They wait for their own parents to die first, they worry about what the grown children might think, they fear they won't find a new mate." Getting out of a bad marriage and getting into a good one can have a tremendous effect on personal energy.

There's also good news for those haunted by the debris of past shattered marriages. A Golden Year marriage may be the best of all. There is some evidence that "bonds between people in their 60s and 70s tend to be the most successful of all. This is because the couples are more mature and the expectations are more realistic. False expectations are what kill many young marriages," says Dr. Stub.

Love Lights the Morning

No one's quite sure how it started, but sex and nighttime have been linked since day one. It probably has something to do with hiding our naked bodies in the darkness. It's time to shed a little light on lovemaking.

"Sex can be an energizer. I see no reason why people only do it right before they go to sleep," says psychoanalyist James O'Hagan, Ph.D., of Manhattan. "Sex is a great way to start the day. The feelings will linger, and it puts you in a good mood."

quently than married men, and unmarried women 10 times more frequently than married women, notes Dr. Lynch.

Those who live alone spend on the average 13.5 days in a hospital for a given illness; married individuals spend only 8.5 days hospitalized for the same illness, says the National Center for Health Statistics.

"All things considered, marriage is society's masterpiece. Those who nurture love in marriage are potentially the happiest lovers of all," writes Dr. Allan Fromme in his book.

BEDROOM BOREDOM

If you've noticed there's one marital (and nonmarital) problem area we've deftly avoided, give yourself a point. It is, as Ann Landers calls it, "The Act." If you're still not catching on, the original three-letter word is sex. Ann created quite a stir in 1985 when she asked her legions of female readers what they preferred, to be held and cuddled, or "The Act." When an astounding 72 percent of her nearly 100,000 responses said they preferred to forgo "The Act," it set off weeks of counterresponses from doctors, psychiatrists, psychologists, other columnists—you name it. *Chicago Tribune* columnist Mike Royko gave his male readers a chance to respond. He found that while most were satisfied with their sex lives, a highly vocal minority were anything but. A number of men preferred trips to the dentist to sex with the wife, while others preferred bowling.

Those who scoff at Ann Landers's unscientific survey, take note. The *New England Journal of Medicine* disclosed that in a study of 100 happily married couples, 50 percent of the men and 77 percent of the

women reported a lack of interest or excessive anxiety about sex. And those were the happy couples!

So what's the big turn-off of marital sex? Tiredness, in both body and soul.

"Fatigue is an important element in the involution of male sexuality and exerts an ever-increasing influence during and beyond middle age," assert famed sex researchers William H. Masters, M.D., and Virginia E. Johnson. Surprisingly, the researchers report that physical fatigue from recreational activities deflates the sex drive worse than job-related fatigue.

Masters and Johnson add that mental fatigue, such as "occupational, financial, personal and family emergencies," takes an even greater toll. Add the middle-age staples of alcohol and excessive eating and it's no wonder so many fires go out.

"Without a doubt, one of the most common complaints I hear from couples in their late twenties and early thirties is they're too tired for sex," agrees Shirley Zussman, Ed.D., past president of the American Association of Sex Educators, Counselors and Therapists. Stress, sprinkled with job, kids, sports and clubs, is the fatiguing factor.

"Couples are investing sexual energy at the job or even at the gym. It's a turn-on to be good at your job or sport. But by the time you get home, you're ready to collapse. After a day of appointments, sleep may seem more tempting than getting excited. These days, sex competes with sleep," Dr. Zussman says.

In two-career couples, the fatigue can be multiplied. "If both partners have jobs, children and a full life, they absolutely have to plan ahead.

They have to establish priorities, and sex is certainly one," says James O'Hagan, Ph.D., a psychoanalyst from New York City.

Husbands, listen up. "If a woman in a two-paycheck marriage is liberated the way women are liberated in Russia—they go to work and then they come home and take care of all the household chores, too—then that resentment can come out in the bedroom," Dr. O'Hagan warns.

When fatigue is caused by untreated illnesses such as anemia, hypothyroidism, diabetes, or circulatory problems, the sex drive can be the first victim.

Although hypothyroid victims enjoy sex when they get around to it, "frankly, they would rather sleep," confirms Isadore Rosenfeld, M.D., author of *Second Opinion*. Curing or treating the illness can have the added benefit of restoring the sex drive.

If these or other ailments are complicated by fatigue-inducing medications, more water douses the sexual fires. Common antihistamines, tranquilizers, antidepressants, ulcer medications, blood pressure drugs, diet pills and, in an ironic twist, even birth control pills can have you reaching longingly for your pillow instead of your mate. Likewise, drinking coffee and smoking cigarettes may kill desire.

The cures for most of the sexual problems mentioned here are reminis-

Is There Love after Sex?

We frolicked through the sexual revolution of the 1960s. We've learned the "joy of sex." We've lost our "fear of flying." We know "everything you always wanted to know about sex" and are no longer afraid to ask. We've become one sexually satisfied nation! What? Hold that last statement. Psychologists (and Ann Landers) say we're still as sexually lost and unsatisfied as ever, if not more so? What gives? Our priorities, respond psychology professors James Halpern, Ph.D., and Mark Sherman, Ph.D., of State University of New York.

In their book *Afterplay,* the two men say we've ignored the most vital aspect of sex, the crucial intimate moments after sex, when so many of us roll over and conk out. Roll back around and listen up. Dr. Halpern and Dr. Sherman found a nation of people lusting for cuddles and sweet nothings instead of postsex snoozes. They found that lovers need to continue the moment in another form. The most popular ways were gentle touching, loving words, conversation, mutual relaxation, privacy and quiet, soft lights and music, a change of surroundings, bathing together and sharing food and drink. Some mood killers you absolutely should avoid following the big moment are leaving immediately, ignoring your partner, rushing off to wash, reading or watching TV, arguing, criticizing, making comparisons or having detailed discussions of performance.

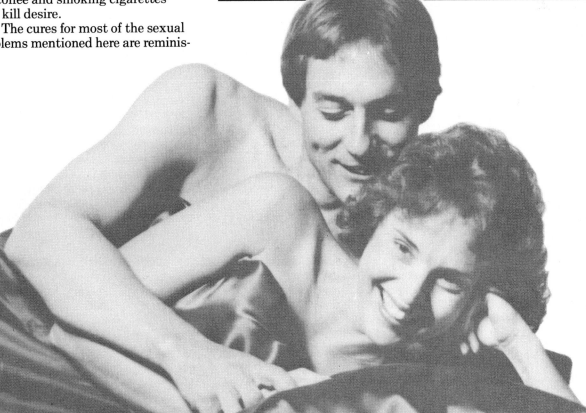

The Vitamin E Fallacy

Sorry, guys, but that vitamin E you pop to energize your sex life isn't doing the trick. If you were a rat, a cricket or a microscopic pond denizen, you'd be in luck. "It was a natural progression to relate the sexual effect of vitamin E on these animals (it improved their fertility) to humans, but that just hasn't been the case," says James R. Litton, Jr., Ph.D., explaining how the wildly popular myth began.

Dr. Litton, a professor of biology at St. Mary's College, Notre Dame, Indiana, and a vitamin E researcher, says if a man believes the vitamin will turn him into a sexual superman, it psychologically could manifest itself in better performance, "but physically, it's not doing a thing for them in bed."

cent of an old medical joke. "Does it hurt when you do this?" the doctor asks, raising the patient's arm. "Yes," screams the patient. "Well, don't do this," decrees the healer.

In short, don't bring the job into the bedroom; overtire yourself in other activities; allow dual careers to keep you apart; let stress strip your desire; let energy-sapping illness go untreated; or allow unspoken resentments to ice the blood.

If these cures are easier read than done, here's more concrete help.

A sensible daily exercise program can increase energy, improve appearance, aid circulation, reduce stress, lift performance, boost self-confidence and, for men, increase levels of testosterone.

PAYING THE PIPER

Maybe sex isn't your problem at all, at least not directly. It's reaping what you sowed that's bleeding your energy. Nobody told you what a bushel of fatigue that bundle of joy really can be.

Someone should have. The entire process of bearing and raising children is one in which fatigue will be a constant companion.

"There's no worse enemy during labor than fatigue," warns *The Pregnancy after 30 Workbook*, giving a good indication of what's to come. And what's to come is more fatigue. "Rest and sleep are vital for the new mother. You must learn to nap and take advantage of whatever rest periods you have during the day."

Introduction of one small child into the home roughly doubles the amount of time a woman spends in domestic activities. And it's usually Mom who suffers the brunt of child-rearing fatigue.

"Most men have little idea of how much time goes into domestic work; they seem to believe that the cleaning gets done by elves in the middle of the night," says Susan Washburn, Ph.D., author of *Partners*. Dr. Washburn and other experts suggest sitting down and organizing a plan that allocates responsibilities, not just between husband and wife but among the other children as well.

In essence, give Mom a break!

As the child/children mature, the fatigue merely changes. Often it shifts from physical to mental, with a good chunk finally landing on Daddy's broad shoulders.

"In our youth-oriented consumer culture, children have their own cereals, radios, alarm clocks and illustrated underwear; they have bras at 10, Princess phones at 12 and automobiles at 16," comments Anthony Pietropinto, M.D., co-author of *Husbands and Wives*. "In addition to providing these luxurious necessities out of the family budget, parents are expected to ensure that their children wind up in more prestigious professions and higher income brackets than their forebears." Dr. Pietropinto offers some sobering statistics regarding the cost of child-rearing. It has rocketed from a positive factor of "100 [English] pounds of financial profit in terms of labor" in 1776 to a conservative cost of $100,000 or more in today's world (other estimates have put the cost closer to $200,000, based on leaping higher education costs).

Because of this frightening financial drain, the current trend is to hold off on having children until later in life. Aside from the stress and trauma of playing "Beat the Biological Clock," this can lead to another example of shifting, but not eradicating, the fatigue. An older couple may not have the vigor needed to nurture active young children.

Before blindly following the latest TV talk show technique on computer-age parenting, let's glance back into the past. Expert theories on eased discipline may have added to the emotional, mental and physical fatigue of modern child-rearing. Many experts now admit the once-praised permissiveness of the 1960s and 1970s, aimed at unchaining the child's creative impulses, lead instead to what one psychologist describes as "parents in paralysis of will," enslaved by "abusive, destructive and manipulative children." Seems the old saying was right all along in its "spare the rod, spoil the child," advice. Just make sure the rod is used in love, not in anger, frustration or jealousy, or as an outlet for your own emotional problems.

DON'T BEAT 'EM, JOIN 'EM

An innovative way of handling the tiring effects of children is to join them in their fun and games. Their "all play, no work" lifestyle may counter yours perfectly. One father found that joining his four-year-old daughter on the playground consisted of climbing up and down a sliding board, swinging vigorously, bouncing across monkey bars and a "grueling 10 minutes of deep knee bends on the seesaw." He concluded that the fun-filled afternoon gave him a better workout than his normal morning and evening jogs. And no doubt his daughter was thrilled.

For those wrestling with the $64,000 question of whether, in today's nuclear world, they should have children at all, Dr. Washburn says it best: "Parenthood is by no means essential for a rich and meaningful life, nor does it automatically introduce a new stage of maturity, but it does provide some exquisite joys, and pains, not to be found in other human experiences."

GETTING AWAY FROM IT ALL

Vacations have been with us from the beginning. In the opening of the Bible, God had barely finished creating the planet when he took a vacation—a one-day break. We've kept that tradition, added another day and crowned it with the title "weekend." Modern society added even more time—the two-week vacation. This is to the year what a weekend is to the week, a time to refresh the body and soul.

But watch out. Some vacations can be as tiring as your regular workday routine and leave you worn and frazzled instead of refreshed. The word *vacation* conjures up such positive images that few people associate it with the killer fatigue that can result from jet lag, overeating, overdoing, stress, cramped family quarters and a host of other nightmares.

"For people who don't know how to handle their leisure time, vacations can be a disaster," warns recreation studies professor William

(continued on page 82)

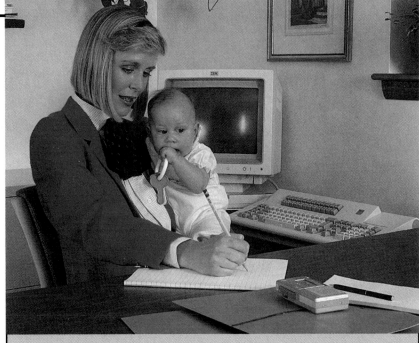

Success and the Supermom

She danced through the TV ad as Enjoli perfume's perfect woman. Irreplaceable executive, devoted wife, ideal mother, gourmet cook, pristine housekeeper. She was Superwoman! She was also, according to experts, supertired.

"Some women are successfully pulling it off, but for every woman who has combined these roles in a realistic and satisfying manner, there must be a hundred who have not," says Marjorie Hansen Shaevitz, a marriage and family therapist and author of the book *The Superwoman Syndrome*. The most common physical symptom, she says, is fatigue. "More and more I hear about women pushing themselves to the point of physical and/or psychological collapse."

Other symptoms Ms. Shaevitz details are dizziness, headaches, pain or tension in the neck, heart palpitations, nausea and muscle spasms. And these are just a few of the physical symptoms. One expert paints the real version of the sweet-smelling Enjoli lady as being unappreciated and suffering from "the Joan of Arc syndrome—the person is being burned at the stake while she tries to make everyone happy."

Ms. Shaevitz believes Superwomen should apply the brakes a bit and realize no one is perfect. She offers commandments such as: don't surrender all your time to others; don't try to do everything; learn to say no; attend to your needs; delegate responsibilities; give loved ones priority; and focus on the positive.

TV and Fatigue

The TV Lobotomy

What happens to your brain waves when you watch "Gilligan's Island" and other titillating TV fare? Psychologists at the Australian National University at Canberra call it a mental version of sleepwalking. As your eyes focus on the TV, they say, your brain waves slow down into a preponderance of alpha and delta brain waves. That's their way of saying the brain goes on automatic pilot, meaning no organized thought is possible in these states. Surprisingly, this brain pattern seems to hold whether you're watching "The Smurfs" or "60 Minutes."

One professor cuts through the jargon and says the brain is "spaced out," and adds, "instead of training active attention, television seems to suppress it. Television trains people only for being zombies."

Four hours a day. That was the average American TV diet in 1978. Then technology kicked in. Suddenly, we were dazzled with 100-channel cable systems complete with 24-hour all-sports and all-music broadcasts. Huge antenna dishes and video cassette recorders plunged in price, enabling regular folks to cart them home to feed their new stereophonic TVs. Many who had nearly abandoned television were enticed back. The result: average daily viewing time soared to nearly 7 hours—or almost half your waking day!

Toss in the hours spent mastering video games and home computers, and a fitting new word has been coined—vidiots.

But vidiot refers only to the brain drain. What is all this glassy-eyed, small-screen viewing doing to our bodies? Making energy as obsolete as cathode ray tubes, according to national fitness expert Charles T. Kuntzleman, Ed.D., author of *Maximum Personal Energy*.

"When you become hopelessly addicted to the role of a spectator, you deny yourself the opportunity to be your own stimulating, energizing agent," he says. "You have, in effect, declared, 'I can no longer find energy in things that I do, only in things that I sit back and watch.' The result is a pervasive form of boredom that typifies nonenergetic people.

"There is nothing inherently wrong with a soap opera or situation comedy," Dr. Kuntzleman adds. "There is something drastically wrong, however, when that show becomes a fix, mainlining a quick kick to us to get us through the day. Whenever we have to go outside of ourselves for stimulation, we lay ourselves wide open to negative addiction, which could lead to decreased energy. A lifestyle dominated by television viewing can hardly be described as energetic."

ANTIADDICTION ADVICE

Jerry Mander, a high-powered New York advertising executive turned antitelevision crusader, calls the deenergizing effects of television "dimming out the body."

"While we are watching television, our bodies are in a quieter condition over a longer period of time than in any other of life's nonsleeping experiences" says Mander. "The heartbeat slows to idle, the pulse rate tends to even out. Viewing positions are chosen in which arms and legs will not have to be moved," he reports in his controversial book, *Four Arguments for the Elimination of Television*.

Doctors and fitness experts say such stilling of the body vastly decreases the flow of energizing oxygen. The result is listlessness.

If you're watching TV more than 2 to 3 hours a day, weaning yourself from the tube can do wonders for your vitality. Here's help:

- Is your television the center of attraction in your home, perched like a god upon an altar? Does all the furniture face it? Put it in an out-of-the-way place. If you make it an effort to watch, you'll be surprised how many programs aren't worth the effort.
- Break TV's "hypnotic spell." Exercise during the commercials by running in place or doing push-ups or sit-ups. Jog around the block between shows or during station breaks. Make it a family game to see if you can return before the show begins.
- Do you really *need* three TVs, or even two? Do a little video cleaning around your house.
- Never flip the switch just to watch what's on. Plan your viewing in advance. When the designated shows end, shut it off.
- Throw the remote control out—or at least hide it in the back of the closet!

What do you do with all the free time once TV is no longer the center of your evening entertainment? Roll off the couch and try some of these reenergizing alternatives.

- Participate! Walk, run, bike, swim. Take up a fun-type exercise or take up a hobby. Build a model or cabinet. Visit a roller rink or bowling alley. Join a softball league or local health club. *Do anything.*

- Create! If you have an unused talent, use it. Take piano lessons, paint a picture, sharpen your photography.
- Activate! Take a course at your local community college, attend your city commission meetings or get involved in church or community activities.

BOOB-TUBE BABYSITTERS

Turning TV off to you also means turning it off to the kids—even if TV provides the opportunity for some peace and quiet. Television shouldn't be a babysitter. Experts say most programs not only expose children to a bombardment of questionable advertisements but also can dull the mind, stifle imagination, induce poor reading skills and may ignite aggressive behavior.

In addition, TV has long been described as an electronic pusher of horrible eating habits.

"When you take a child who sits and watches television from the age of 2 to 10 or 11 and sits in front of the Saturday morning TV box and listens to sugar, sugar, sugar, sweetness, sweetness, sweetness, chocolate, chocolate, that child picks up a habit which is going to continue through life," said a leading television critic testifying before the U.S. Senate.

A study by Fran Matera, Ph.D., of the University of Miami, concluded that up until age five, children can't even distinguish between the programs and the advertisements. In their world, Sugar Bear and Tony the Tiger teach as effectively as Sesame Street's Big Bird and Kermit.

In light of this growing concern, many parents have limited their children's viewing to a single hour each night, while others have invoked a total blackout on week nights. Increased exercise through active play usually results.

(For more on children, TV and fatigue, see "The Tired Child Syndrome.")

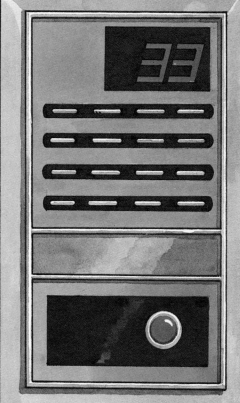

The Tired Child Syndrome

Has your kids' get-up-and-go got-up-and-went? Is poking a button on a remote control device their most energetic endeavor? If so, they could be victims of "the tired child syndrome," caused by an overdose of television.

In a study of 30 chronically fatigued children, Richard M. Narkewicz, M.D., and Stanley N. Graven, M.D., discovered that all were heavy TV watchers—3 to 6 hours on weekdays, 6 to 10 on weekends. Sleep and appetite disturbances, altered behavior, anxiety, headache and abdominal pain often accompanied the fatigue. The doctors discovered that TV intoxication is a "self-perpetuating cycle" resulting in fatigue and illnesses that limit children's activities to watching even more television.

They prescribed a total TV boycott. They also ordered "vigorous physical activities" after school and quiet recreational activities in the evenings. The results were that the "blacked-out" children began improving in 3 to 7 days, and lost all symptoms within 2 to 3 weeks. Other children, who watched on a limited basis, took longer to recover.

In a follow-up study, the doctors found that 11 of 13 children who returned to unrestricted boob-tube-dominated lifestyles were again suffering from the same symptoms.

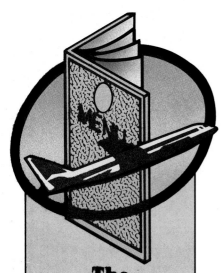

The No-Jet-Lag Diet

Jetting? Here's a diet to beat jet lag. If traveling eastward, eat well three days before. Eat light the second day (low-calorie, low-carbohydrate foods). Feast again the day before. Eat light the day of the flight. Start liftoff day with a high-protein breakfast. Drink coffee or tea without sugar or milk while flying. Skip the airline fare. Sleep. Avoid alcohol. When you arrive, eat a big lunch and dinner. Go to bed early.

If heading westward, follow the same plan but drink additional coffee or tea during the morning of your flight, and none after noon.

Theobald, Ed.D., of Purdue University. "So many adults, especially working couples, cave in to the kids' demands on a vacation and ignore their own needs and desires."

Dr. Theobald suggests gathering the troops and holding a family conference prior to planning the trip. If the fur starts flying, University of Minnesota family social science professor Paul Rosenblatt, Ph.D., suggests separate vacations may be the cure, although this should be the last resort. For example, if Dad's and the boys' idea of Nirvana is a mosquito-infested fishing camp, Mom and the girls can opt for Disneyworld. Families that must remain a unit can choose a diverse resort where everyone can do their own individual thing.

If the conflicts can be resolved, or family isn't a factor, Dr. Theobald suggests finding out who you are before you decide where to go. Comfort-oriented people should steer toward less exotic spots that offer "all the comforts of home," and in turn avoid the stress and fatigue of severe culture shocks. Adventurous types can shoot for the exotic places or one-with-nature vacations.

"Often it is the antithesis of work that turns out to be the most leisurely," Dr. Theobald advises. "If your job is sedentary, you might enjoy an active vacation. If your work is physically demanding, a week of lounging at a resort may be best."

FITNESS VACATIONS

A popular trend in today's health-oriented society is the fitness vacation. This is a broadening of the idea of the old sports-oriented vacations—skiing, surfing, diving, swimming—that are geared to allow everyone to participate. They can range from simple walking tours of Japan or other foreign countries to treks through the wilderness areas of the western United States. Other examples of such invigorating getaways that can be reserved with a simple call to your travel agent include:

- Horseback or bicycle riding through France's Loire Valley.
- Backpacking through New Mexico's historic Pecos Wilderness and Sante Fe.
- Climbing Mt. Fuji in Japan.
- Rambling along the Cornwall coasts of England and Wales.
- Strolling through German, French, Italian and Romansh (native Swiss) neighborhoods, all within a hearty walking distance in the same country—Switzerland.
- Hiking the famous Long Trail of Vermont, going from rustic inn to rustic inn.
- Charting the great rhododendron forests as you climb the Himalayas of Nepal.
- Rowing 100 miles down Utah's glorious Green River Wilderness.
- Canoeing "North America's Last Great Wilderness"—Canada's Northwest Territories teeming with vast herds of caribou, white arctic wolves, moose and grizzlies.
- For those who like to "go American," a similar wilderness canoe adventure through the Allagash Wilderness Waters in northeast Maine.
- Or any number of bicycle tours through such places as New York's wine-making Hudson Valley, the Inca trails in Peru, or Lake Michigan's Northeastern shore.

If you have trouble tracking them down, Overseas Adventure Travels, Mountain Travel or Intimate Glimpses are packagers your travel agent should recognize.

Even these active tours can be ruined if your frame of mind isn't good when you start, or if the traveler's bane of jet lag or auto fatigue knocks you out.

If you're a workaholic executive who'll be stressed out by the thought of two weeks away from the job, psychiatrists suggest taking a number of shorter, three-day, extended-weekend vacations instead of one long, anxiety-inducing getaway.

TRAVEL FATIGUE

Jet lag fatigue is a modern affliction caused by jet-setting too fast through the world's time zones. Your normal eat, sleep and work/play routines become topsy-turvy. Arriving at your destination a few days early to adjust or mimicking the sleep/wake cycle of your destination before you leave are two ways to combat it. Eating properly also can help.

If you're driving to your fitness vacation, you certainly don't want to be dozing at the wheel. Here are some helpful hints for keeping your wit—and your energy level—running smoothly on long car trips.

- Take advantage of the roadside rest areas every few hours. Doctors say that taking a "body refueling" break every 2 hours helps you to stay alert at the wheel. High-energy take-along snacks— not fast food fare—are recommended.
- Avoid drugs that cause drowsiness, including allergy tablets, antidepressants, tranquilizers, sleeping pills, motion sickness medications, painkillers, epilepsy drugs or medication for high blood pressure.
- Both driver and passengers should avoid smoking. A buildup of haze on the window can impair vision, causing tired eyes.
- Don't push it. Don't drive beyond your normal sleeping time.

THE ENDLESS SUMMER

If you're gearing up for that eternal vacation, otherwise known as retirement, you should beware of the myriad physical and psychological problems that frequently erupt during this volatile period. Fatigue is the most common symptom. The best way to counter it is to identify the enemy and face it head-on.

The big decision is when, if ever, you should retire. Federal laws, pressure groups such as the Gray Panthers, social attitudinal changes and better health have pushed a number of retirement ceilings to 70. Some people feel even that is too low.

"Having any mandatory retirement age is cruel and unusual punishment," says Gordon Fuqua, M.D., a psychiatrist and family therapist at Michael Reese Hospital in

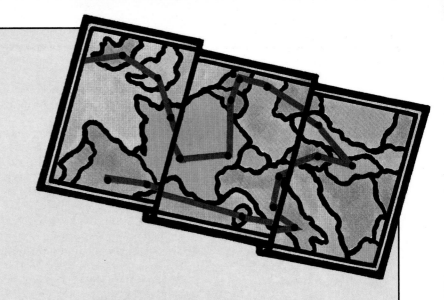

If It's Tuesday . . .

Considering one of those popular European "sightfleeing" jaunts, the kind that inspired the farcical movie *If It's Tuesday, This Must Be Belgium*? These whirlwind romps, designed for folks who demand the most from their vacation buck, are not for the faint of spirit or body.

"The main problem is they are relentless. There's just no time to relax," says tourism professor John Schroeder of Purdue University. Consider a recently advertised 17-day wonder tour that encompasses England, France, Switzerland, Italy, Austria, Germany, Holland and Belgium. That's only the countries. The trip includes pit stops in 19 cities and bedding down in 11 different hotels! The blur of sights ranges from St. Paul's Cathedral in London to St. Mark's Basilica in Venice.

Or, how about this schedule for day 14—blast off from Mannheim for a Rhine cruise from St. Goar to Boppard, dash to Cologne for a snapshot, then sprint to Amsterdam, Holland. Day 16 launches your worn-out body from Amsterdam to Belgium, where it's catapulted to Calais, France, then lobbed to London.

If this sounds like your kind of trip, ask yourself a few tough questions. Are you physically up for such a blistering pace? Do you intend to drag along a spouse, child or friend who can't keep up? "The fatigue can be awesome," Schroeder warns. Before reserving your spot, a full physical examination and consultation with your doctor is a must. Let good sense prevail. As your American Express tour guide might say, "Don't leave home without it!"

Chicago (and a mere babe of 45). "I think it is ageism, akin to racism. Those decisions should be made on an individual basis. I don't intend to jump in a rocking chair at 65."

Unfortunately, not all employers agree. And a countertrend today is to offer inducements and bonuses for early retirement to bring "fresh blood"—i.e., lower salaries—into the company. If you're persuaded to "voluntarily" retire, doctors say the important thing is to see it as your gain and the company's loss.

"It's crucial to think young," Dr. Fuqua says. "A lot of the problems of people getting older are based on cultural expectations. They say you can't dance anymore, you can't have sex, you can't be athletic, you can't work. You're supposed to sit on the porch and rock. It's absolutely untrue. But there can be a self-fulfilling prophecy to that. The people who do well are the ones who don't stop for anything, who maintain the same interests, social circles and hobbies. It's vital that you stay active in all the areas that we humans demand for a vigorous life."

Staying physically active is emphasized by virtually every doctor and gerontologist consulted. Study after study has confirmed that exercise and active lifestyles can slow the ravages of aging. And these studies are backed by studies showing that people are staying healthier as they grow older, with life expectancies closing in on 80 for both men and women. If you take a bonus retirement package at age 55, that means you have a full quarter century to enjoy life!

So enjoy. Too tired? You've just gotten into some bad habits. Reenergizing your golden years is as simple as learning to walk.

Equal Opportunity Retirement

He's retired. Now you have to make lunch as well as breakfast and dinner. He's living the life of Riley, while you're still pre-prince Cinderella, cooking, washing, ironing and scrubbing. No fair! This is the nightmare of the everyday housewife who finds that the double standard lives on after hubby calls it a career.

"I can understand women becoming bitter if her husband's work ends, but hers hasn't," says Chicago psychiatrist Gordon Fuqua, M.D. "If this is a problem, I would recommend negotiations to share the tasks. This may free time for the couple to do things together. It may also help a lost husband with nothing to do."

Dr. Fuqua says there are additional retirement problems along the same line. The executive husband who suddenly decides to become "boss" of the house and starts barking orders can drive any woman batty, while "just having the husband underfoot, like he's another child to rear, can be difficult." Delegating chores equally and encouraging the man to take up outside interests can ease the transition. If the tyrant syndrome occurs soon after retirement, don't reach for the rolling pin. Dr. Fuqua says it may be a temporary period of adjustment. A sympathetic spouse can opt to wait it out. High-energy exbosses usually move on to more challenging endeavors.

LIVE LIFE TO THE VO₂ MAX

J. L. Hodgson, Ph.D., a physiologist at Pennsylvania State University, says one of the keys to energy is "maximum oxygen consumption," or VO_2 max. It declines steadily with age, starting at 30. Unlike most aspects of aging, it can be rejuvenated. Hodgson says a 70-year-old on a moderate exercise program can increase his VO_2 max to a level equal to that of someone 15 years younger. Exercise up to an athlete's level can turn the clock back a whopping 40 years!

"There is no drug in current or prospective use that holds as much promise for sustained health as a lifetime program of physical exercise," agrees Walter Bortz, M.D., of Palo Alto, California. It's a medicine so potent another researcher has called it the closest thing to an antiaging pill.

Senator Alan Cranston, 71, the force behind the establishment of the

National Institute on Aging and a contender for the Democratic presidential nomination in 1984, attributes his youthfulness to a regimented exercise routine.

"Without my current running, I know I couldn't maintain the pace that my Senate responsibilities demand," he says.

Is Cranston an exception? Only in his dedication to exercise.

"For millions of people, getting older means getting more tired," says Herbert deVries, Ph.D., an expert in gerontology and professor emeritus at the University of Southern California. "But the real culprit is not age. It's a body so unused to activity that it tires at the slightest effort."

In addition to reviving energy, exercise has proven to invigorate the cardiovascular system, improve skin tone, lower blood pressure, increase joint flexibility, restore muscle tone, firm up sags, strengthen bones and reduce varicose veins. The type and level of exercise for you depends on your current condition. Generally, doctors recommend three 30-minute sessions per week of aerobic exercise, including walking, cycling, swimming, jogging or racquet sports. Consult your doctor before starting.

If mental fatigue's got you down, exercise can pump energizing oxygen to your brain.

"The human brain does not shrink, wilt, perish or deteriorate with age," says British gerontologist Alex Comfort, M.D. Exercise keeps the mind honed by increasing reaction time, short-term memory and reasoning power.

Nutritious diet should team with exercise for a lifetime daily double. A Pritikin-type diet (we say "Pritikin-type" because his diet is needlessly overstrict), high in complex carbohydrates and fiber and low in fat, salt and cholesterol, is a good place to start. In fact, Nathan Pritikin has now proven its effects beyond question. After his death at 69 in early 1985, a complete autopsy was ordered. Doctors found his arteries to be "amazingly clean for a man his age." Stephen Inkeles, M.D., of Santa Monica added, "Pritikin had the arteries of a pre-adolescent boy." Free blood flow is vital to energy, especially as you get older.

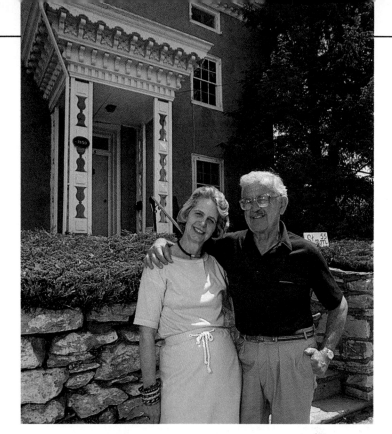

Renovated Lives

For 35 years, Bill Storm was a reporter on the mean streets of Philadelphia. He wrote about murderers and heroes, cops and robbers, the gifted and the desperate. It was a fast-paced, exciting life. When it was gold watch time, Bill Storm, like many people, found it hard to grind to a halt. His solution? A second career—a growing phenomenon in the 1980s as people retire healthier and live longer.

Bill, 68, and his wife Jean, 55, teamed up to refurbish a 135-year-old, 3-story house in the historic Quaker town of Plymouth Meeting, Pennsylvania, a few miles outside Philadelphia. In 6 months, they transformed a "wreck" into the beautiful Bell Portico, a bed-and-breakfast inn. "I couldn't just sit around and do nothing. How many novels can you read?" Bill says, downplaying his efforts. "Having this work to do motivated me. I'd get up at 6:00 A.M., sand the floors, paint the walls, do some woodwork, then collapse into bed at 11:00 P.M." Adds Jean: "It's wonderful to see an old room bloom into something beautiful. There's a tremendous amount of satisfaction in that."

Although Bill says he "worked so hard people were telling me to go see a doctor" his doctor probably would have sent him back to work. Physicians say second careers can renovate a tired, fatigued life as well as a building.

7

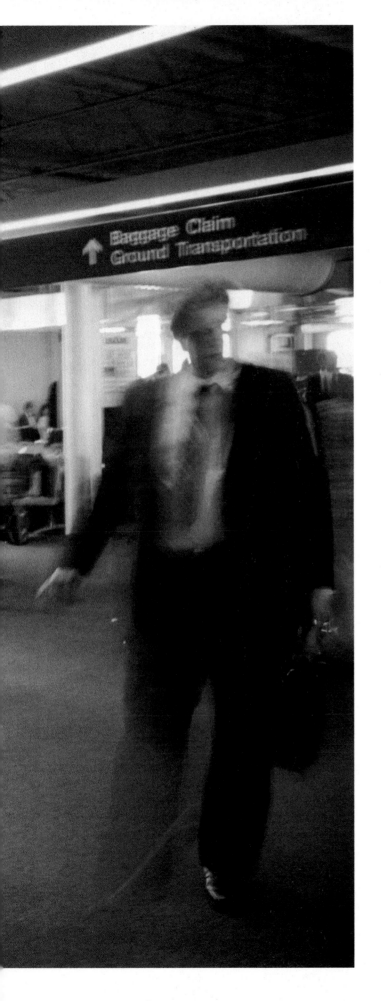

Learning to Manage Your Time

If you make your minutes count, you can bank on having a more rewarding day.

I f, like songwriter Jim Croce, you could "save time in a bottle," you would never be late for a plane, a train or a bus. You would be on time for all your appointments and ready for every big date. It would be truly wonderful if you could call on time like some magic genie whenever you needed it.

But time, which some consider even more precious than gold or diamonds or oil, cannot be saved in bottles or barrels or vaults. Time cannot be saved at all. It can only be spent. And the key to getting the most value out of your time is to spend it wisely. This is what time management is all about.

By managing your time wisely, you can increase your energy level and use your energy more efficiently. And the first step toward doing that is to realize that your energy level is influenced not only by your mental and physical health but also by the time of day. As discussed in chapter 4, each person's body has its own built-in clock that is attuned to the 24-hour turn of the earth. Your energy level is controlled in part by your internal clock, or circadian rhythms, as this phenomenon is called.

Some people bound out of bed in the morning with their personal energy batteries fully charged, ready to roar down life's highway at full throttle. These same people may start to run out of gas by midafternoon and about an hour after dinner they're exhausted and ready for bed.

Other people have a terrible time getting out of bed in the morning. They start the day on four flat tires, bumping over an unpaved road. But these slow starters often are ready to shift into overdrive when the sun goes down. While the early risers are nodding off to sleep in front of their television sets, the night people are putting on their sneakers or dancing shoes and heading off to

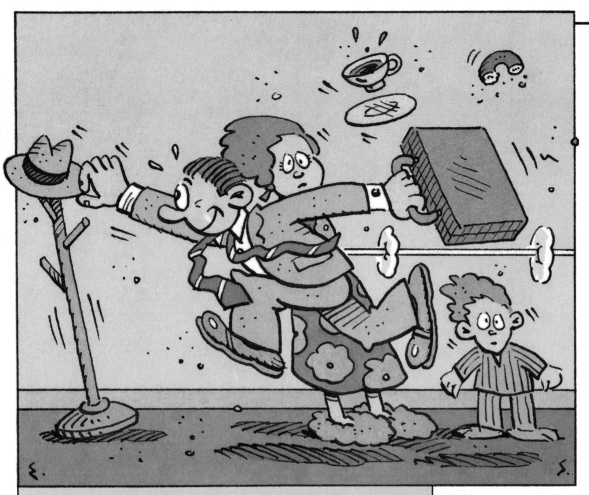

Beat the Clock to Work

Tony and Robbie Fanning, authors of *Get it All Done and Still be Human,* say the secret to being on time is to give yourself permission to move up your deadline. Tell yourself you must arrive at work at 8:45 instead of 9:00 A.M. and aim for that deadline. You probably will be late as usual, but when you arrive at 8:55, you will still be 5 minutes early for work.

play racquetball or to dance the night away at the local disco.

Both types of people have the same amount of energy. They just have it at different times of the day. Scientists estimate that two-thirds of the population of the United States is made up of "day people" and one-third of "night people."

To increase your energy level, you have to figure out which category you fall into. Then you should schedule your most taxing activities at the times when you're most energetic. This way you can be most active when your energy level is high and avoid struggling through periods of low energy. Ask yourself the following questions:

- Do you feel good when you wake up?
- On weekends or vacations, when do you go to bed and when do you wake up?
- What is your happiest time of the day?
- What time of day do you feel the lowest?
- What time of day do you like to make love?
- When is your biggest meal?

Your answers to these questions should indicate to you when your energy is up and when it is down. The next step is to train yourself to use your energy-charged moments to your best advantage.

PRIME TIME FOR THE JOB

Ken Cooper, Ph.D., who lectures on how to increase personal productivity, describes in his book *Always Bear Left* a survey he gave to 2,000 working adults. Dr. Cooper asked each person to rate his or her productivity or alertness on a scale from 1 to 10 on an hourly basis from 7:00 A.M. to 6:00 P.M. The survey showed morning start-up was slow. Attentiveness was best in the period from 9:00 to 11:00 A.M. People crashed shortly before lunch as fatigue overtook them. They started up again slowly only to come down again in late afternoon. The best performance of the afternoon was scarcely better than the worst showing of the morning, Dr. Cooper's survey showed.

"The scheduling requirements are obvious," Dr. Cooper writes. "People require light, early warmup to get the neurons flowing. The midmorning is best for heavy thinking requiring high attention or reactive listening. Breaks should be more frequent as lunch approaches—and never work past noon! The afternoon should be kept lighter, possibly filled with physical activity or interpersonal communicating. The late afternoon hours are largely a waste and overtime is productive foolishness."

As an example, he cites a secretary who spent 2 hours typing a report one afternoon, then retyped the same report two mornings later in 1½ hours. "She felt she was working just as hard each time," Cooper said, "but the second time she was typing at a more productive time of day. Without realizing it, she had wasted ½ hour the first afternoon."

FIRST THINGS FIRST

Planning your workday and the workdays of your employees to make the most efficient use of your time and their time is one of the keys of good time management. R. Alec Mackenzie, a time management expert and author of *The Time Trap,* retells the story of how Charles Schwab, during his days as president of Bethlehem Steel Corporation, learned

a valuable lesson from consultant Ivy Lee. Schwab told Ms. Lee, "Show me a way to get more things done with my time, and I'll pay you any fee within reason."

Ms. Lee handed Schwab a sheet of paper and said, "Write down the most important tasks you have to do tomorrow and number them in order of importance. When you arrive in the morning, begin at once on number 1 and stay on it till it's completed. Recheck your priorities, then begin with number 2. If any task takes all day, never mind. Stick with it as long as it's the most important one. If you don't finish them all, you probably couldn't do so with any other method and without some system you'd probably not even decide which one was most important. Make this a habit every working day. When it works for you, give it to your men. Try it as long as you like. Then send me a check for what you think it's worth."

Weeks later, Schwab sent a check for $25,000 to Ms. Lee with a note saying the advice was the most profitable he ever had received.

Quite simply, if you set your priorities this way, the most important things get the most attention and your least important tasks get set aside until you have time for them.

So take the time to plan each day. Decide what your priorities are and write them down. It might help if you keep in mind the Pareto Principle, which later became known as the 80/20 Rule. Vilfredo Pareto, a 19th-century Italian economist and sociologist, came up with the theory that the largest percentage of the value of a group of items is contained in only a small number of the items.

Life is filled with examples of how the Pareto Principle works. Twenty percent of any sales force accounts for 80 percent of all new business. Eighty percent of all television viewing time is spent watching only 20 percent of the programs. Twenty percent of the students in a class take up 80 percent of the teacher's time. The principle often is applied to the workplace. It is generally conceded that 80 percent of any manager's time is taken up with nonessential tasks. Most managers accomplish their most productive work in just

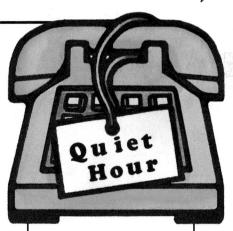

Sh-h-h—It's Quiet Hour!

Some companies have designated a "quiet hour" to provide an uninterrupted period of concentration for their employees. At a Michigan insurance company, these are the quiet hour guidelines: no outgoing phone calls, no paging, no unnecessary talking, no excessive movement.

More than 90 percent of the employees find their concentration and organization improve when they are not interrupted. Some managers found the hour so profitable they added a second quiet hour a half-hour after lunch.

20 percent of the time they spend on the job.

THE MEETING MUDDLE

Rita Davenport, a time managment consultant and author of *Making Time, Making Money,* has some tips for getting the most out of one of the biggest energy zappers in the working world—business meetings. When holding a meeting "make sure you *start* on time, *stop* on time and have only *key people* in attendance," she stresses.

"Another tip is to hold short, informal meetings standing up," Ms. Davenport says. "When I was a schoolteacher I suggested we test this theory by holding our next faculty meeting standing up and then measuring the results. The meeting lasted only 12 minutes, 33 minutes shorter than the previous meeting. And we still covered all the essentials." She found that what was eliminated was the idle chit-chat, cigarette smoking and coffee drink-

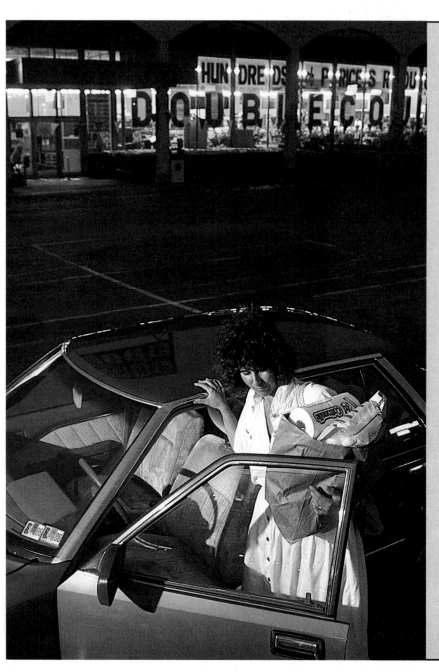

Living Off-Peak

Avoid the maddening crowds that take up time and test your temper with just a tad of planning.

- Avoid the lines for the 7:00 P.M. movie by going to the 5:00 P.M. show and then going out to dinner.
- Buy your Christmas cards in January. You'll save money, too!
- Reserve your tennis or racquetball courts for 7:00 A.M. or after 10:00 P.M.
- Shop through mail-order catalogs and avoid the crowded shopping malls.
- Ship your Christmas presents to faraway relatives by ordering them through catalog companies that will mail them for you.
- Go to lunch at 1:30 instead of 12:30 P.M. It's easier to get a table and to have your meal served promptly.
- Visit Europe in the winter when the rates are cheaper and the tourists are gone.

ing that usually interfered with
the meetings.

HOUSEWORK—THE BEST APPROACH

We now live in a world filled with
modern conveniences that were not
even dreamed of two decades ago, yet
it seems some people never have any
time to enjoy themselves. They always
have too much work to do, either at
home or on the job.

Philosopher Bertrand Russell, in
his essay, "In Praise of Idleness,"
points out that we have used our
technology to make twice as many
pins in a given time instead of the
same number of pins in half the time,
which would increase the time we
have to relax and enjoy the fruits of
our labor. Russell complains: "There
was formerly a capacity for light-
heartedness and play which has been
to some extent inhibited by the cult
of efficiency. The modern man thinks
that everything ought to be done for
the sake of something else and never
for its own sake."

In short, we don't make any time
for fun and enjoyment. And we
should. But there's the job, and the
house and the kids and the car and
the . . . Where do you begin?

Just as you set priorities to
accomplish work on the job, you also
should set some priorities for your
work at home. This includes such
things as housework, yard work,
errands—all those unpleasant tasks
that are necessary to make our lives
livable but that we wish we could live
without.

Most people get into set habit
patterns in which so much of their
time is allotted for their job and so
much for household tasks (which are
really just another form of work).
Whatever time is left over is for
pleasure. Unfortunately, that isn't
always enough time.

So, following the logic you follow
for your job, make a list of just what
you want done and how often you
want it done. Do you want to vacuum
once a week? Twice a week? How
about dusting? How much of that
does your house *really* need? Dishes
have to be washed every day, but

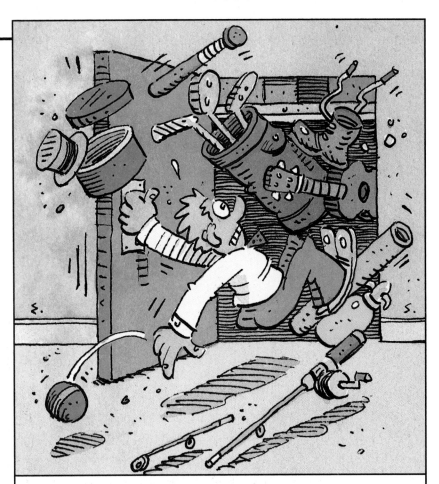

Let's Get Organized!

The best way to keep track of your belongings so
you don't waste time looking for them is to have a
place for everything and have everything in its
place. This does not mean you should pitch
everything into the nearest closet. That's the
out-of-sight, out-of-mind system of filing—everything
is out of sight and you're out of your mind if you
think you can find it.

A better way to organize all the cupboards and
closets in your home is to make a list, giving a
rating of 1 to the most convenient, easy-to-reach
spaces and a 10 to the places that require a ladder
or a deep knee bend to reach. Next, make a list of
your stored belongings and rate them from 1 to 10,
depending on how often you use them. Your
everyday dishes, for example, should be in a handy
cupboard. Your Thanksgiving carving set should
be tucked out of the way.

If you find you have too many number 1 items
and not enough number 1 storage space, it's time to
put up more shelves or cupboards or hang a
pegboard with lots of hooks on it.

Flex-Time Saves Time

In the 1970s the federal government started a new policy that allowed workers to start their 8-hour day a couple of hours earlier or later. A study of 30 U.S. agencies on "flex-time" found 83 percent less tardiness, 71 percent less absenteeism and short-term leave and longer hours of service to the public.

The study also found employee morale 86 percent higher due to more job satisfaction, easier commuting, easier child-care arrangements and better control of the employee's own time.

that's what automatic dishwashers were made for. Once you've completed your list, break it down into days of the week with different chores listed each day. Set a time to dust, a time to vacuum, a time to toss the laundry into the washer and dryer. Then do each appointed task at its appointed time. Set a timer. When it goes off, stop. In their book *Get It All Done and Still Be Human,* Tony and Robbie Fanning suggest you should never allow work time (housework, that is) to interfere with fun time and that you should always do your fun activities first. "We know a woman," they write, "who works full-time but who is also a budding songwriter. Meanwhile, she lives in a house which gets annoyingly dirty. Every night when she gets home from work, she writes songs or reads or listens to music until midnight, at which time she spends an hour cleaning house. She never allows housework to interfere with her songs because, as she says, 'I can clean the house when I'm tired from writing songs, but I can never write songs when I'm tired from housework.' "

Some people get up early and do their housework before breakfast. Others prefer to let it go all week and then work like crazy on the weekend. Find the time that's right for you. Just make sure it doesn't take up *all* your time.

There is probably no group of people who experience energy drain more than women who are trying to juggle a career and a household at the same time. "Women are trying to be all things to all people, and they become victims of circuit overload," says Robert Eliot, M.D., internationally renowned stress expert, author and clinical professor in the University of Nebraska's department of preventive and stress medicine.

An antidote for overload that Dr. Eliot prescribes for his patients is to "take some personal time—maybe 20 minutes a day—to do something selfish. Don't treat yourself like a robot."

If you don't think you have time, *find* time. "Reorder your priorities." Dr. Eliot says. If that means dinner is served at 7:00 instead of 6:00, so be it.

Fran Nelson, director of the

Parental Stress Center in Madison, Wisconsin, offers these suggestions for working mothers to find time to reenergize. Other women also can benefit from the first three and single fathers can benefit from all of them.

- On your way home from work, take several long, slow, deep breaths, "It really does help reduce tension in the body," she says. Spend twice as much time exhaling as inhaling to prevent hyperventilation. Be aware of the tense places in your body and imagine that you are breathing deeply to them.

- List the things you want to accomplish each day and forget about the items at the bottom. Maybe a spotless house isn't the most important thing.

- "I don't think I can stress enough that everybody has to have time alone—to read the paper or just relax," Ms. Nelson says. "Get your fair share, even if you have to go into the bathroom to get it." Make that clear to the children. "Reading the newspaper is my big event," she adds.

- If you have school-age children, telephone them from work as soon as they get home from school. That way, they'll communicate the exuberance of their day to you then and won't have as much of a need to pounce on you when you arrive home. Ms. Nelson says this technique works well for her—she's a single parent of three teenagers.

- Don't feel guilty about saying no. If your child wants you to do something you really dislike, you can usually substitute something you'll both enjoy. "I do not blow up balloons," she says, and her children know it.

- Give the children jobs around the house, especially at mealtime. That way, she says, "everyone feels like a part of the whole," and you have more energy to do things you enjoy.

A SPACE FOR YOURSELF

Working mothers seem to agree unanimously that combining demanding careers with chores and the pleasures of parenthood is the greatest challenge they face.

"The hardest thing is making time for yourself personally," observes Ricky Arce, a mother of two who commuted more than 2 hours to and from law school where she was a full-time student.

"I've quit reading novels and doing needlepoint," she said. "I've given up taking pictures, fixing up the family album and writing letters. I've lost track of a lot of people. Things I used to do leisurely, like shopping, I now do as quickly as possible. But on the positive side, I nag the kids less. I make fewer demands. I used to be a little compulsive. I've gotten more relaxed. Plus, it's nice to have an excuse not to do the things I *don't* like to do— like housework."

Washington lawyer and mother Linda Kay Davis seconds that sentiment. "I abhor housework," she says, "so having an excuse to hire someone is terrific." With two young sons and one poodle, she and her husband, Bob, both of whom are supervisory trial attorneys with the U.S. Department of Justice, share the trials and rewards of their hectic lifestyle.

Linda and Bob must use their lunch hours for their personal recreation— her dance classes and his racquet sports. After work they head straight home to relieve the babysitter. Although they often took traveling vacations before they had children, they now find such trips expensive and logistically difficult— and energy draining.

"My house is not as neat as my mother's house, but then I've never

(continued on page 98)

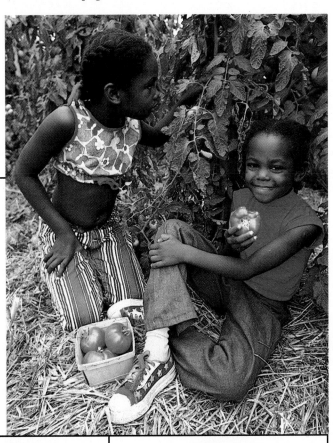

27 Chores That Kids Can Do

You delegate authority at work, so why not delegate authority at home? Get the kids to pitch in with the household chores. It'll give you time to do other things you want or need to do. Children can become household helpers at a very early age. Reward them for the work they do, either with an allowance or a special treat. It'll give them a feeling of accomplishment—and of being needed.

5- to 8-Year-Olds

Pick up clothes and toys. Answer the phone. Feed the pets. Walk the dog. Make the beds. Dust the furniture. Set the table. Clear the table. Get the mail.

9- to 12-Year-Olds

Wash the dishes. Empty wastebaskets. Take out the garbage. Vacuum. Wash windows. Weed the garden. Make school lunches. Clean their room. Do errands.

13- to 16-Year Olds

Mow the lawn. Wash the car. Dig the garden. Do the laundry. Cook meals. Wash and wax floors. Trim hedges. Paint the house. Wax the car.

Time in Other Lands

Attitudes toward time vary widely from culture to culture. Industrialized countries such as the United States, England and Germany are obsessed with the clock. "Punctuality has become a virtue that we demand of those around us," says economist Staffan B. Linder, author of *The Harried Working Class.* "Waiting is a squandering of time that angers people in rich countries. . . . They are haunted by their knowledge that the shining moments are passing without things having been done." This is a far cry from how people in other cultures view time.

JAPAN

People in Japan are not dominated by the clock. Their work and leisure activities fall into haphazard patterns. Japanese office workers think little of putting in extra hours at their jobs without pay if they are asked to do so. They don't always eat at the same times of day. They are very casual about appointments and guests may show up early or late. Everyone is expected to have a flexible schedule that can be adjusted easily.

GREECE

Greeks pass time rather than budget it. In most villages, peasants leave for the fields at dawn and return home at sunset. At night they visit and chat in their homes or local coffee houses. There is no set time for Mass on Sunday or for dinner. You go to church and eventually the service begins. When you are invited to dinner you are expected to come and visit—eventually dinner will be served. This has changed in the cities, but Greeks still bridle at the idea of watching the clock.

LATIN AMERICA

People in poorer countries where productivity is low have extra time on their hands. They have no great need for sticking to a time schedule. In these cultures you will find a *mañana* attitude—there's no big deal about what must take place today, because there is always tomorrow. In fact, they are so blasé about time that the "rush, rush" concept of busy, industrialized countries is even hard to translate into their languages.

MIDDLE EAST

People in the Middle East also have a relaxed view of the passage of time. Edward T. Hall, author of *The Silent Language*, says with Middle Eastern people, "it is pointless to make an appointment too far in advance, because the informal structure of their time system places everything beyond a week into a single category of 'future,' in which plans tend to 'slip off their minds.'" The Nuer, a pastoral people living in the Anglo-Egyptian Sudan, don't even have an expression in their language equivalent to time.

ALASKA

In traditional, non-Westernized settings, Eskimos live only for the moment. Explorers who first encountered Eskimos living in the frozen Arctic were taken with the fact that the Eskimos lived their lives entirely in the present without much thought to the future. If they killed a caribou, they would sit down and eat it immediately and think little of saving any of it for later. When traveling by dog sled, they would not hesitate to stop for tea, if so inclined, even if a blizzard was raging around them and the village to which they were traveling was only 2 hours ahead.

NIGERIA

When anthropologist Paul Bohannan studied the Tiv people in Nigeria, he noted that the concept of time was very difficult to translate for them. The Tiv kept track of time on the basis of natural phenomena or social events instead of within a chronological system. He found that "although Tiv indicate time by direct association of two events and though they count recurrent natural units such as days, markets, moons and dry seasons, they do not measure time."

Procrastination

Procrastination—sometimes referred to as "the art of keeping up with yesterday"—can seem to be a cute, harmless foible. We all put off unpleasant tasks from time to time. If we're lucky, the unpleasant tasks disappear and are replaced by pleasant tasks. But by procrastinating constantly, we can wind up living an unfulfilled, boring life in which none of our goals is ever met.

"There are a lot of people out there . . . who live with a sense of fraudulence and anxiety because they can't seem to get hold of their procrastination," says psychologist Lenora M. Yuen, Ph.D.

"Time lost in procrastinating can take years out of a person's life," adds William J. Knaus, Ed.D., psychologist and executive director of the Fort Lee Consultation Center in New Jersey. "It saps enormous amounts of energy, emotion and time."

Procrastination is worse than simple laziness. Dr. Yuen maintains that procrastination "is a complex psychological problem that rarely yields to simple remedies."

To really understand how you procrastinate, you have to take a hard look at the little lies you tell yourself when you put off doing things. Dr. Knaus believes those little lies are really expressions of inner turmoil of two basic types— self-doubt and "discomfort dodging," or a low tolerance for tension and frustration.

"Self-doubt is a crippler of action," Dr. Knaus says. "And people who habitually put things off are almost always self-doubters, always asking themselves, 'Should I or shouldn't I do this or that?' "

Dr. Knaus explains that self-doubters "mistake doing the best they can for doing the best there is." And since nobody can do the best there is every time, they end up doing everything late—or never.

Discomfort dodgers, Dr. Knaus explains, procrastinate because they're afraid of the anxious or uncomfortable feelings they associate with starting a task. They put things off to avoid feeling bad. Since everything you try to do in life is bound to produce its tensions and frustrations, he explains, discomfort dodgers are chronic avoiders, shrinking from anticipated pain.

So what can you do to get things done? Dr. Yuen suggests you start by drawing up a list of the excuses you use to put things off. Keep a daily log of your antiprocrastination campaign in a notebook. What types of things do you tend to put off? Is there a pattern? Are all the things you avoid really important to you at all?

But becoming aware of the ways you procrastinate is only half the battle. "Some of my patients have all kinds of insights about their problems," says Dr. Knaus. "They understand them better than I do. Yet they're still at square one." Self-awareness by itself is not enough. There comes a time when you have to act.

Many procrastinators fail to start a project unless they are convinced they will have enough time to finish the whole thing. They value the complete task, not the many steps that lead to completion. Management consultant and author Alan Lakein suggests trying what he calls the "Swiss cheese" approach. Instead of taking on the entire project at once, Lakein advises "poking holes" in the work by taking whatever time you have to do one small part of the overall task. That way, it's easier to get started, you learn to consider each half-hour's work an accomplishment, and you may eventually even complete the job. Here are some other tips to help get yourself started.

- Dr. Yuen says procrastinators tend to think in "global terms" about work; instead of aiming to put the storm windows in by November 15, they vow to "save money on energy." Make your goals specific and observable, and divide the steps needed to get there into small, achievable tasks.
- Whenever possible, Dr. Knaus suggests, develop the habit of doing it *now*, as soon as you think of it, rather than simply adding it to your list of things to be done.

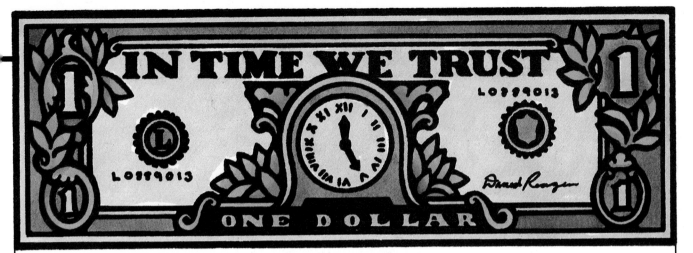

Time Is Money

"Waste your money and you're only out of money, but waste your time and you've lost a part of your life," says Michael LeBoeuf, author of *Working Smart.* "Few of us would knowingly take half of our take-home pay and spend it on something that was of absolutely no use to us or anyone else. However, the vast majority of us spend at least 50 percent of each day in various pastimes that provide no earthly use or satisfaction for anyone, including ourselves. We literally waste away half of our lives and do it in oblivious indifference."

If you live 77 years, your lifetime will consist of 28,124 days or 674,982 hours. That amounts to about 40 million minutes or 2.5 billion seconds. This chart, based on 244 8-hour workdays, shows just how much *your* time is worth in dollars and cents.

If Your Yearly Earnings Are	Every Minute Is Worth	Every Hour Is Worth	In a Year, One Hour a Day Adds up to
$ 2,000	$.0170	$ 1.02	$ 250
2,500	.0213	1.28	312
3,000	.0256	1.54	375
3,500	.0300	1.79	437
4,000	.0341	2.05	500
5,000	.0426	2.56	625
7,000	.0598	3.59	875
7,500	.0640	3.84	937
8,000	.0683	4.10	1,000
10,000	.0852	5.12	1,250
12,000	.1025	6.15	1,500
14,000	.1195	7.17	1,750
16,000	.1366	8.20	2,000
20,000	.1708	10.25	2,500
25,000	.2135	12.81	3,125
30,000	.2561	15.37	3,750
35,000	.2988	17.93	4,375
40,000	.3415	20.49	5,000
50,000	.4269	25.61	6,250
75,000	.6403	38.42	9,375
100,000	.8523	51.23	12,500

Reprinted by permission from *Working Smart: How to Accomplish More in Half the Time,* by Michael LeBoeuf. Copyright 1979, McGraw-Hill.

- Once you have your work momentum going—say, by reorganizing your kitchen cupboards—transfer that energy to another project, like writing a long-neglected letter. You'll probably find it's easier than starting later from ground zero.

- Use what Dr. Yuen's colleague Neil Fiore calls an unschedule. First, determine how much time you've already committed to your regular responsibilities; what remains is unscheduled time that can be thought of as the maximum amount of time you can afford to devote to other projects. As a way of rewarding yourself for steps taken along the road to completion of those projects, note each half hour of work on your unschedule only *after* it has been completed.

And keep in mind that those who can but don't must give way to those who cannot but try.

been as neat as my mother," says Linda.

What are you living for, if not to get some enjoyment out of life? Too many people are so busy earning a living and fixing up their homes and cars that they never have any time to have fun.

We need to take time out from our work—both at home and on the job—so that we can recharge our batteries. Different types of leisure activity work for different types of people. "Some people are action oriented, some are mental," says Beverly Potter, Ph.D., management psychologist and author of *Beating Job Burnout*. She's quick to add that you shouldn't feel you have to be doing something all the time. Tell yourself, "Hey, it's all right for me to do nothing. If I feel like sitting for a while and staring at a wall or lying in the yard and getting a suntan, that is my due. I don't have to be busy all the time." Rewinding can only give you energy to do something better later on.

Tony and Robbie Fanning also note the time famine which keeps many people from having enough time to enjoy themselves. They raise the question of how much of your "free" time actually is free.

It takes time to maintain your own body, to feed it, wash it, groom it; it takes time to maintain your family, especially if there are younger children in it; it takes time to maintain a home (cleaning, laundering, repairing, building, trimming); it takes time not much different from "work" time to do all of these things. It takes time to shop for time-saving

Have Fun with Wasted Time

"Life is on the high-wire," circus performer Karl Wallenda once said. "All the rest is just waiting."

But with a little planning, all that time you spend waiting doesn't have to go to waste. You actually can have fun with it and accomplish a lot of things you normally would not have time to do.

Airports and bus or train terminals are fine places to read novels or to knit sweaters. Planes, trains and buses are perfect settings to write novels or poetry or to catch up on your correspondence. If you live only a few miles from work, you can use commuting time as exercise time by jogging or bicycling instead of driving.

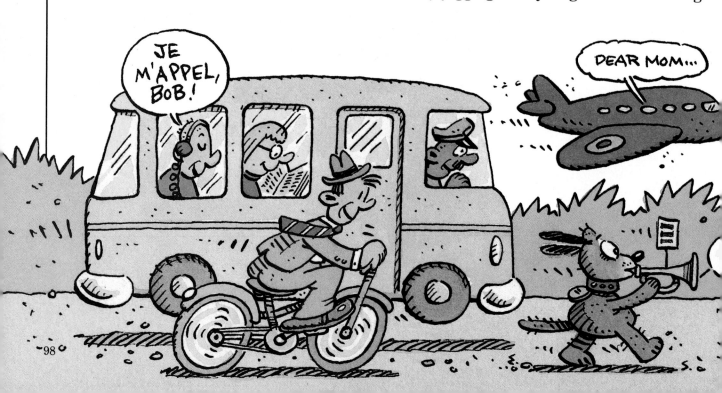

devices; it takes time to use them; it takes time to maintain them; and, in an ironic twist, it takes time to "enjoy" them. All of these are forms of "pseudowork."

Quite simply, if your entire life is run by a make-more-work-for-yourself-than-necessary attitude, you won't have any energy left to do the things you enjoy — the things that make life so worthwhile. But it's not all hopeless. Here are some tips to fit more leisure — and, at the same time, more energy — into your life.

- Draw up a wish list and make sure you follow it. Set some goals. Include some leisure activity, whether it be exercise, playing an instrument or working on a hobby.
- Take a personal time inventory. How do you spend your time? How do you want to spend it? If there's no time for the things you *want* to spend your time on, it's time to change things around — or read this chapter over again.
- Make a time log and see how much time you spend trying to achieve your wish list. If finding time is a struggle, you know you're doing something wrong. Change the way you spend your time so you can achieve your wishes.
- Make a list of the time wasters in your life (like spending hours on the phone) and get rid of them; make a list of time savers (like shopping by mail) and make good use of them.

It's your life. Make sure you have the energy to live it up.

If your commute is long, make the most of it. A Philadelphia publishing executive taught himself French by listening to instructional tapes in his car during his 3-hour daily commute. Another commuter used the time his car was stopped in traffic or at red lights to practice playing a fife.

Tony and Robbie Fanning, authors of *Get It All Done and Still Be Human* say, "We know a man who takes a city bus to the train, rides 30 miles to his work city, and walks the last mile to work. He finishes reading a novel every other day on the train and feels great from walking."

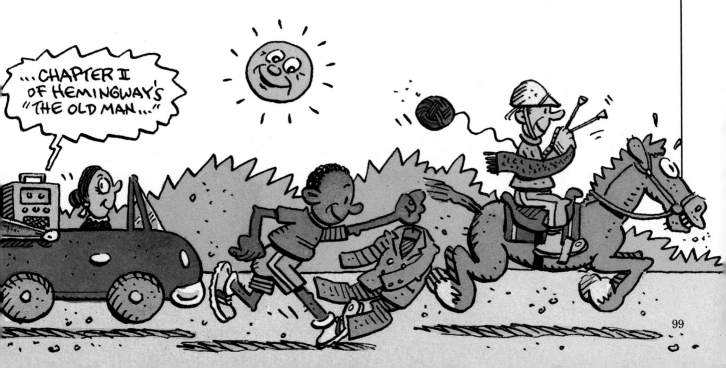

Your Personal Time Inventory

Are you in control of your time? Or is your time controlling you? To find out, do a personal time inventory. List all your weekly activities and classify them into groups as illustrated below. Estimate how much time each activity takes and how much it deserves. Keep a weekly time log as illustrated on page 101 and see how much time you actually spend on each activity. Where did you go wrong? How can you improve? Good planning and management can take time but it's worth it in the end.

Be honest when you analyze your activities and the amount of time you spend on them. Then examine the things that are taking up too much time. What time-wasting activities can be reduced? How many can be eliminated? Can you get someone to help? Are other people wasting your time? What percentage of your goals did you fulfill? Do you spend enough time on the things that are really important to you? If not, why not?

Job Activity	Time It Deserves	Time It Takes
1.		
2.		
3.		
4.		
5.		
6.		
7.		
8.		
9.		
10.		

Personal Activity	Time It Deserves	Time It Takes
11.		
12.		
13.		

Family Activity	Time It Deserves	Time It Takes
14.		
15.		
16.		
17.		
18.		
19.		
20.		

Weekly Time Log										
Time	Mon.	Tues.	Wed.	Thurs.	Fri.	Sat.	Sun.	Activity		Total Hours
7:00 A.M.										
8:00 A.M.										
9:00 A.M.										
10:00 A.M.										
11:00 A.M.										
Noon										
1:00 P.M.										
2:00 P.M.										
3:00 P.M.										
4:00 P.M.										
5:00 P.M.										
6:00 P.M.										
7:00 P.M.										
8:00 P.M.										
9:00 P.M.										
10:00 P.M.										
11:00 P.M.										
Midnight										

Design your inventory around your waking day. How much time do you spend working? How much time do you spend around the house? How much time do you have to yourself? If you make an honest inventory and evaluation of how you spend your time, you'll easily be able to spot areas that need improvement. Make a 1-week inventory and analysis of your time every 6 months. Regular inventories can help you keep track of your progress or the lack of it. Alert yourself to bad habits before they become ingrained and hard to break.

8

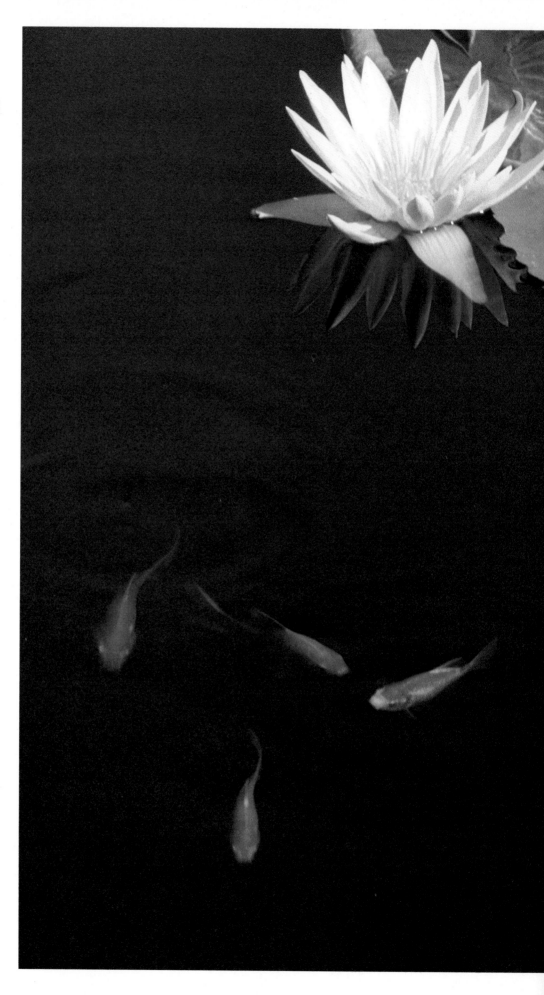

Relaxation: Pathway to Renewal

Stress can sap your energy and your health. But you can arrest this vitality bandit with easy, fun techniques.

Serenity. Calmness. Relaxation. Peace. In the modern world, fewer and fewer of us seem to have even a vague idea of what those words mean as we rush from homes to cars to jobs to stores. Too often "peace" ends up meaning sitting exhausted in front of the TV, watching yet another dreary show, depressed because we have no energy for anything else. And when we finally push the button to turn the screen off, we don't feel refreshed and renewed. We feel drained, like something more has been taken from us.

Our national addiction to slumping in front of the TV is only one symptom of the immense toll the stress in modern life is taking on us. Most of us admit we feel it. In one large survey, more than 80 percent of the people questioned felt they were experiencing too much stress. Only 18 percent said they felt little need to reduce stress.

Does this mean we're becoming a nation of wimps who can't stand the pressure? No. The evidence is in and has been in for quite a while. Stress is no minor inconvenience—it's a modern plague, cutting us down like the Black Death that roared through Europe in the Middle Ages.

If that seems too extreme, consider these facts. Current estimates are that 80 percent of visits to doctors are for stress-related disease. Thirty-seven million Americans suffer dangerous high blood pressure, much of it stress related. One and a half million of us have heart attacks each year, and more than one-third of that group die. Each year, another two million Americans get stomach ulcers. Nine million (some estimates are higher) are alcoholics. Stress also has been linked to cancer. Evidence mounts all the time that stress is tied to the breakdown of immunity.

And this list is only the beginning of our stress-related wounds. To combat stress, we also

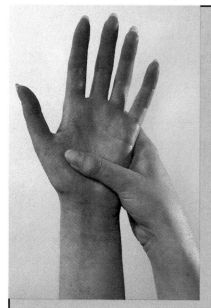

Miracle Massage in Minutes

You usually massage *with* your hands, but you can also massage your own hands to get a mental sense of calm within minutes, promises Phoenix psychologist James McClernan, Ed.D., an expert on stress management.

Hands are an excellent vent for nervous tension because they are virtual extensions of the brain, some researchers believe. And hand massage can be done anytime, anywhere. Here's what to do:

1. Sitting with your hands in your lap, make tight fists. Hold for a count of 5. Repeat 5 times.
2. Press your fingertips together like a spider on a mirror. Press hard, then relax, 10 times.
3. Use your thumb to rub deeply into the palm of the opposite hand, paying special attention to the muscle at the base of the thumb. Massage the webs between thumb and fingers firmly. Rub until each hand is warm and relaxed.
4. Let your hands hang at your sides and shake them. Rub them together briskly.

fill millions of tranquilizer prescriptions and swallow tons of aspirin every year.

STRESS IS EVERYWHERE

So what is this stress that drags us out, saps our energy, clouds our lives and turns health into sickness?

What it's not is your mother-in-law moving in, the extra assignment from the boss, your kid losing her bike or not enough help with the housework. Those are the *stressors,* say the experts.

In fact, when scientists talk about stress, they may be talking about a reaction to happy events, too. Getting married. Getting promoted. Moving to a bigger house. Our bodies can react to these things in nearly the same way as if we got divorced or fired or our house burned down. Our emotions might be different, but the physical reaction is much the same, though it varies in intensity.

Even that wonderful vacation you've planned all year may provoke stress, say experts. And many of us will admit that the first day away from the routine is difficult. In short, *any* change tends to provoke stress.

In one well-known study, investigators rated various life events based on how much stress they produced. Death of a spouse and divorce had expectedly high scores. But so did a new job. The amount of stress accumulated during a year, the researchers found, was an accurate way of predicting susceptibility to illness as well as the likelihood of being involved in an accident.

But other research suggests it's not the big traumas but the little, continuously annoying things—the dripping faucets of life—that take the biggest toll on our energy and our health.

In one study of a group of policemen, it was not their involvement in situations of extreme danger that taxed them. It was their routine frustration over what they saw as unfair coverage by the press and an inefficient legal system that wore them down.

TENSION—HEALTH ENEMY NO. 1

Let these little things get to us too often and we have a tension-filled life. Every little annoyance seems like a big deal. Someone teases you about your electric blue shirt and you snap back. Your friends are suddenly talking about *you*—"Boy, is he in a bad mood." That's because stress has a tendency to build on itself until our reactions are totally out of proportion to the actual source of stress at a particular moment.

Extreme examples are the Vietnam veterans who suffered from post-traumatic stress disorder. Though safe at home in America, they were unable to stop whirling on imaginary enemies, even when only mildly startled. They were just too tense.

More personally, you can see how a decreased tension threshold (psychologists refer to it as a low arousal level) works in your own life. Just think of how you might react to the same event on a good day or a bad day.

If, for instance, little Tommy breaks a treasured heirloom on the day you just got back from a wonderful family vacation, you might feel compassion for the child, take him in your arms and tell him it's okay.

But if the same thing happens on a day when your car broke down, the grocery bag split and Tommy came home with a row of D's on his report card—well, we won't speculate on how you might treat poor Tommy.

Psychologist George S. Everly, Jr., Ph.D., co-author of *Controlling Stress and Tension*, compares our arousal level to the idle of a car. "If it goes too fast, we burn out our motor. But we can set it lower and still have plenty of energy when we want to step on the gas," he says.

Tense people burn too much energy, warned the late Edmund Jacobson, M.D., in *You Must Relax*, an early classic on the subject. But you can learn to control tension and increase your stores of energy for the time you really need them. How? By learning how to relax.

TURNING DOWN THE PRESSURE

When we're relaxed, our heart and breathing rates slow, muscles ease and blood pressure dips. We feel calm—in control. We're in a state that is helpful rather than harmful to our energy and health—the opposite of stress.

Relaxation has the ability to turn off tension. We aren't pacing because the bus is late, or irritated by loud noise, grumpy people and the myriad other stressors of our times.

By learning how to relax for as little as 10 minutes a day, you can lower your stress level and feel more energetic.

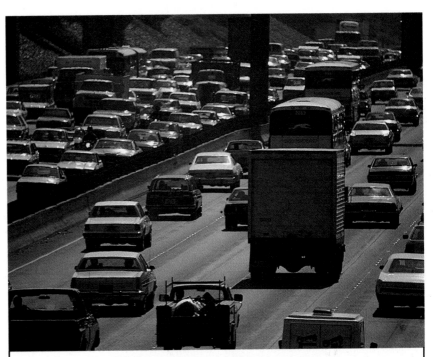

Emergency Relaxers

Cruising off the cloverleaf, you see it—a trophy-worthy traffic jam. You feel tension knot your insides like a classic Boy Scout clove hitch.

In this or any other stress-soaked situation, take the heat off and release that agonizing tightness with one of these quick emergency stress relievers recommended by the experts.

Fantasize. Take a mental jet to your favorite vacation spot. Or graciously accept the Nobel Prize.

Sing. A bellow, a lilt or a dirge, singing calms you and helps you vent feelings honestly.

Pray. If you're a doubter, pray to Whomever It May Concern. Or use prayer to see what might be there.

Breathe Deeply and Slowly. This is a time-honored cure for tension or fear.

How it all works is still a mystery to scientists, although clues emerge all the time. Whatever the reason, scientists are convinced that relaxation is the key to handling stress. Unfortunately for many of us, relaxing is something that doesn't come easily. (Picture the co-worker who always looks frazzled.) But, say the experts, it can be learned. And by learning a few relaxation techniques, you can control your stress instead of having your stress control you.

Most of these life-, health- and sanity-saving relaxation techniques are surprisingly easy to learn and simple to do, although they do require practice. Among the most successful are the techniques that focus on your ability to exert conscious control over your body. These techniques—which, by the way, have been scientifically tested and proven to give long-term benefits—include various breathing exercises, meditation and Progressive Relaxation.

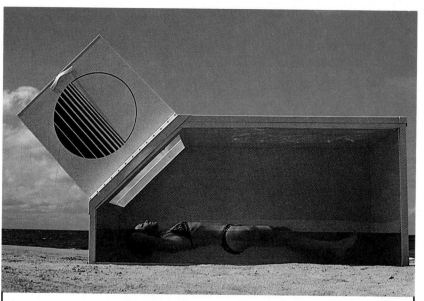

Floating to Nirvana

For those so tense they believe that nothing short of a sledgehammer to the back of the head could relax them, there is the flotation tank—possibly the world's shortest route to deep relaxation.

In a pitch black tank, insulated against sound, you float in a foot of water warmed to body temperature and so supersaturated with Epsom salts that you are virtually weightless. The floating is so effortless, the water so supporting, your muscles refuse to hold tension. Cares seem to float away in the satiny water as breathing becomes slow and regular. You hope the music that ends this peaceful, womblike experience is a long way off. Tanks rent for up to $40 an hour—but the benefits are said to last for weeks.

EASY BREATHING, EASY LIVING

"Take a deep breath." It may have been the first relaxation technique you were ever taught.

When you were a kid and you came into the house crying, so upset you couldn't get the words out to tell your mother what was wrong, that was the instruction she gave you.

You took a deep breath and it worked. (Being held in her arms for a minute or two might have helped a little, too.)

In giving you breathing instructions, your mother was just repeating centuries-old folk wisdom. But it's folk wisdom that's being supported by modern medical journals.

Heart researcher Otto H. Schmitt, Ph.D., was one scientist who accidentally documented the calming effect of slow, regular breathing. In an effort to get an accurate, consistent measurement of heartbeats, he programmed a computer to give people standardized instructions on breathing.

The instructions resulted not only in slowed heartbeats—a sign of relaxation—but in reported feelings of calm. Some subjects became so mellow, in fact, that they fell asleep.

Of course, practitioners of yoga have used breath-control techniques for thousands of years to gain mastery over their minds. They regard the breath as the most important tool available for mental discipline. And lately scientists have come along to raise a rather tardy banner verifying that breath control works.

At the Kripalu Center for Yoga and Health in Lenox, Massachusetts, a major center for the training of yoga teachers, a number of breathing techniques for calming and energizing the mind are taught.

One of these methods is known as breath watching. Just a minute or two of each hour of your workday spent mentally observing your breath as it moves in and out of your nose will keep you fresh and relaxed all day long, promise the Kripalu yoga teachers.

When you watch your breath without making any conscious effort to control it, it tends to fall into a peaceful pattern as your mind becomes absorbed in what your body is doing, say Kripalu experts. Breath watching very simply makes sure that you *are* breathing rather than unconsciously holding your breath, as you may do when stress strikes.

Breath watching, by the way, is a favorite technique of Buddhist meditators who count breaths up to ten, then start again. Supposedly it was this breath-watching technique that Buddha himself was doing on the day of his enlightenment.

YOU'RE GETTING CALMER

How does regulated breathing work to induce calm? Altering the concentration of carbon dioxide in the blood may play a role, say scientists. But breathing also calms in the same way meditation does, mainly by turning your preoccupation with your struggle with the world into the attitude of a passive observer. Many types of meditations, in fact, rely on the rhythm of the breath.

And just like muscle-relaxing methods, controlled breathing sends a message to your brain that you *are* relaxed. Regulated breathing apparently does this by stimulating the vagus nerve, a major part of the relaxation response system that passes through the chest and slows the heart, experts believe.

Relaxation breathing methods also are believed to pacify by feeding back soothing messages to the brain through the Hering-Breuer reflex, the mechanism that normally keeps the air moving in and out without your having to think about it.

Alternate-nostril breathing is one of the most powerfully relaxing and rejuvenating of the breathing techniques. Why use only one nostril at a time? Some experts theorize that switching nostrils somehow activates both halves of the brain—the left, logical side and the right, artistic side—to work in tandem. When that happens, there's a feeling of balance and completeness, of harmony. To do this exercise, use the ring finger of your right hand to control your left nostril and your thumb to close your right. (It's a good idea to blow your nose thoroughly before beginning this exercise.)

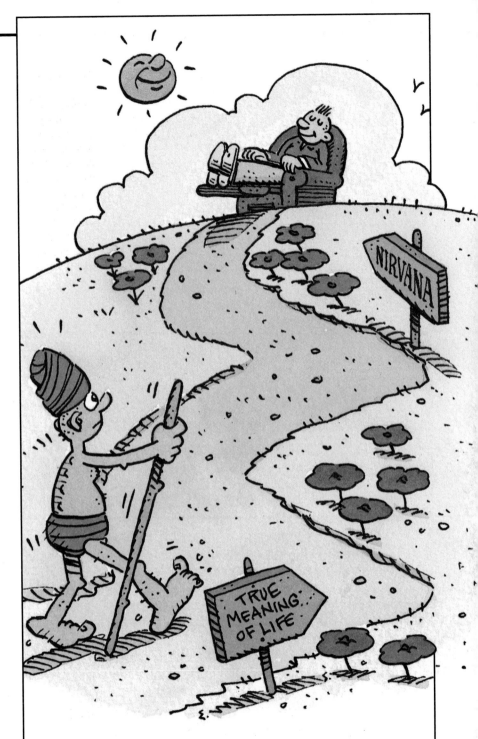

The Easy Chair Way to Inner Peace

Comic strip character Dagwood Bumstead napping on the couch may be approaching bliss as fast as a monk contemplating a lotus blossom. That's the conclusion of University of Kansas psychologist David Holmes, Ph.D., who compared meditation with plain old leaning back in a reclining position. He found the measurable benefits to be exactly the same. Any comfy spot, from the couch to a new $1,600 massage lounger, will do, says Dr. Holmes.

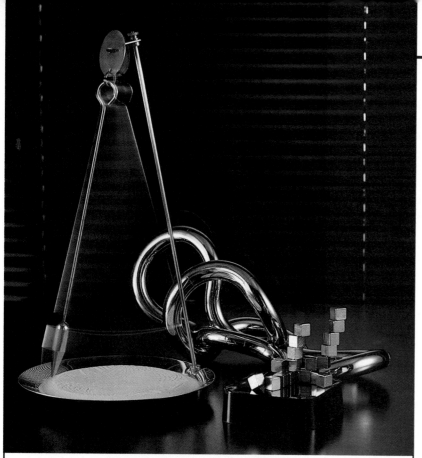

Executive Pacifiers—
They Do the Job

You shouted at your secretary, snapped at a client and hung up on your business partner—in short, you really lost your cool. But before you take your frustrations out on anyone else, why not soothe your frazzled nerves by turning to an executive toy. Such "toys" (there are scores of them on the market) make attractive additions to any office, and they really do offer a "hands-on" solution to calming corporate anxiety.

The CRDL (pronounced *crid-dle*), for example (above right), uses metallic cubes and a powerful magnetic base to unleash creative energy and pacify even the most irate VIP. Mad at your boss? Just sculpt his or her likeness and knock it over. Or stick to fashioning gentle arcs and curves.

Like CRDL, Tangle (above center) moves, bends, twists and shapes itself into an infinite number of forms. Its attraction, however, is the sensuous way it feels—a few minutes of idle sculpting are sure to calm and soothe you.

The Pit and the Pendulum (above left) provides a more passive means of relaxation. Once started, the pendulum swings hypnotically back and forth for 15 to 30 minutes, producing beautiful patterns in the dish of glass beads beneath it.

You can now start breathing in through the left nostril to a count of two. Hold your breath for a count of eight, then breathe out through the right nostril to a count of four. Then breathe in through the right nostril to a count of two, hold for eight, then breathe out through the left nostril to a count of four. Repeat the sequence. You can continue this for as long as you want, but 5 minutes is a good time period.

Pharyngeal breathing, called the Ujjayi technique of breathing in yoga, is another technique that can "calm down the mind," says Fern Marshall, Kripalu yoga teacher. To do it, just relax and breathe in and out slowly and deeply, from the region at the back of the mouth—the pharynx. Keep your mouth closed and your nostrils passive. Make a snorelike noise, particularly as you exhale. As silly as it sounds, a few minutes of this technique can leave you feeling as if you could handle anything.

Plain, deep breathing is one of the most useful of the tension-reducing tools because it can be used anywhere, anytime, explains Ronald Dushkin, M.D., a physician who teaches at Kripalu.

"No one can ever tell you to stop breathing," he says. "As a doctor, I tell you to keep breathing. It's in your best interests," he jokes.

MEDITATE YOUR TROUBLES AWAY

Many scientific studies have shown that the system copyrighted as Transcendental Meditation (TM) works in eliciting the relaxation response with all its benefits, and TM courses are available in most communities. The only drawback is that TM costs about $450 to learn.

Other methods, such as Clinically Standardized Meditation devised by Patricia Carrington, Ph.D., can be learned from moderately priced tapes. And Harvard professor Herbert Benson, M.D., who coined the phrase, "the relaxation response," has a popular book by that name that teaches all the hows and whys of meditation.

But you may find that you need no more than the simple instructions offered here to start reaping the rich rewards of meditating.

Dr. Benson's instructions are simple: Once or twice a day, sit comfortably in a quiet place. Allow your eyes to close. Let all of your muscles relax, starting with your feet and working your way up to your jaw and face.

As you breathe naturally through your nose, repeat a simple word or phrase on each exhalation. Don't worry about "doing it right." If your mind wanders—as it probably will—just let it come back to the word. This passive attitude is the most important part of the procedure, says Dr. Benson. Do this for 10 or 20 minutes. Then just sit quietly for a minute or two before returning to the world.

In *The Relaxation Response,* Dr. Benson recommends "one" as a fine word to repeat during meditation. He has since suggested that additional benefits may be gained from a word or phrase that has personal religious or spiritual meaning to you. Some examples: "peace," "life is a journey," "joy is inward," or "God is love."

THE ABC'S OF MUSCLE RELAXATION

Dr. Jacobson was one of the first Western scientists to link a high and prolonged level of muscular tension to an A-to-Z list of physical and mental disorders. Dr. Jacobson stated flatly that multitudinous modern ills could be prevented or relieved through muscle relaxation.

Mere rest, he said, was not enough for most tense people. Many of us had been tense so long, he said, we'd forgotten what a relaxed muscle felt like. Some of us are even tense when we sleep! (Do you grind your teeth or awaken with clenched fists?)

Dr. Jacobson invented a simple program for learning how to let go of muscular tension. He called it Progressive Relaxation, and it's still widely used today, sometimes prescribed by therapists to tension-wracked patients.

But some of you are saying, "My problem isn't in my muscles! My problem is Junior flunking out of vocational school, Sis running off with the rock band Slime and the

Superstitions Can Ease Stress

Elayne Kahn, Ph.D., knocks on wood and makes wishes on a star.

A scientist with something good to say about superstitions? Yes. Lucky charms and a little abracadabra may be just what we need to ease us through the tensions of the modern world, says the New York psychologist.

"Superstitions relax us because we feel we're doing something to help ourselves," says Dr. Kahn. If you rub your lucky coin before going in to talk to the boss, for instance, you're more likely to go in with a positive attitude, she explains. And because you feel more confident, things are more likely to go well. Using such a charm "gives people a sense of security about the unknown forces in life," notes Dr. Kahn.

And since they're often based on something that's personally meaningful to us—a lucky number from an anniversary date or a lucky piece that's a souvenir of a trip—our superstitions "encourage a sense of belonging in an otherwise alienated world," explains Dr. Kahn, the author of *1,001 Ways You Reveal Your Personality.*

An act like wishing on a star can actually help you toward a goal, says the psychologist. "By expressing a desire, you encourage yourself to fulfill that desire." And both having specific goals and reaching for them are stress reducing.

Superstitions may even help you build stress-easing friendships, she points out, for "people who follow superstitions are people who think about their behavior and are more likely to be thoughtful and considerate of others."

Home-Groan Relaxation

Arrgghhh!! A long, deep groan like that may sound like an expression of pain, but it can be your song of health, says a relaxation expert.

Groaning—a natural, old-fashioned response to physical or mental pain—releases the hurt and tension and allows you to feel better, says Louis M. Savary, Ph.D.

Groaning also relaxes you physically because it forces you to breathe deeply and gives a soothing massage to your internal organs, Dr. Savary explains.

Plan a groaning session of at least 10 minutes, advises the expert, who has taught his method to more than 4,000 people— including nuns who now do "prayerful groaning." Put on cover-up music like wailing jazz, lie on your back and start to groan. Or you can groan in your car on your way back from work. You'll arrive home refreshed, says Dr. Savary.

boss asking me to run the Zoo Fund charity drive on my own time."

You feel like you could care less about what your calf muscle is doing; what you need is to stop worrying about the kids and the gorilla house.

But it *is* what is happening in your calf muscle and the 1,000-plus additional muscles in your body that is breaking you down and wearing you out, leaving you fatigued, listless and prey to disease and accident.

Moreover, because we have the ability to exert conscious control over our muscles, they are an excellent site for throwing the "off " switch on tension and turning on the relaxation instead. And muscle relaxation provides almost immediate relief from tension, both physical and mental. Through a system called the proprioceptive nerves, your muscles inform your brain that they are relaxed, and your brain responds by calming down, too.

NEVER-FAIL RELAXATION

To do Progressive Relaxation, just get into a comfortable position, either lying on your back or sitting. Take a couple of slow, deep breaths, then begin by clenching your left foot. Hold for a second or two, then let it go. Tighten, then relax, your left calf. Work your way up, tightening and relaxing your thigh and hip. Then start on your other foot and work your way up to the top of your head.

Although this and other relaxation skills may seem mindlessly simple, they work. But not without a little trying. Relaxing well—like any physical skill—requires practice. And though Progressive Relaxation will help in a pinch when you're feeling a great deal of pressure, the best idea is to integrate it into your routine when your life is relatively smooth. It will help you stay relaxed throughout the day and help you avoid falling victim to stress.

QUICKIE RELAXERS

But maybe you feel these techniques take too much time, that they create even *more* pressure in a packed existence. Well, here are some meth-

ods recommended by stress-reduction experts that will fit inconspicuously into the most crowded day.

Jeffrey Migdow, M.D., a doctor on the staff of the Kripalu Center and a stress-relief expert, recommends a relaxation technique called an awareness check.

Again, it is simplicity itself. While sitting comfortably, allow your eyes to close. Take one or two deep breaths. You're going to focus your mental awareness on different parts of your body, simply noticing in turn how each part feels—any sensation, tension or relaxation. It's important not to judge how you feel, just observe it. You can bring your awareness first to your left foot. See how your toes feel. Note any unusual sensations. Check your sole.

The awareness check proceeds slowly up your left leg to your hip and buttocks, then starts again with your right foot and continues up to your neck and jaw. Notice if there's any tension there. Let your lips separate slightly. Then simply observe the thoughts in your mind as if they were passing by on a television screen, without judging them. Take a slow deep breath and you are ready to open your eyes. For maximum benefit, make sure you are breathing deeply and regularly.

"Many people become aware of areas of tension they didn't know about," says Dr. Dushkin. "People also notice that those areas of tension are often relaxed after going through this." This technqiue takes only 3 to 5 minutes. And some people teach themselves to do it even while walking down a hall from one meeting to the next.

And if you're really pressed, here's another quick calmer. Called the quieting response, it was invented by a Yale professor. While seated comfortably, allow your head and shoulders to droop gently forward, letting your chin hang toward your chest. Take a deep breath and smile. That's it!

Just smiling itself can help, says Dr. Dushkin. "One of the most frequent prescriptions I write is, 'Smile before meals and at bedtime.' " It's very pleasant to consciously smile, he says, and it may be just the break you need.

PEOPLE NEED PEOPLE

Some things that cause you distress can't be changed—the loss of a loved one or financial problems to which there's no immediate solution.

You do what you can for yourself despite the difficulty. You eat right and continue to exercise and you practice a relaxation technique regularly. Is there anything more you can do to help yourself handle the stress?

Yes, there's plenty. One of the greatest stress easers is simply relating to other people. Someone's shoulder to cry on, someone to laugh with and mainly just someone to listen to you can improve your outlook almost instantly.

Our friends and family help us keep things in perspective and see that our life is bigger than whatever is bothering us. They tell us that tomorrow is another day and that things will get better.

Because they are so stress relieving, family and friends are tremendously good for our health. And it's well known that married people live longer and have fewer illnesses than singles.

Caring human contact is literally lifesaving. One recent study showed that a simple 15-minute how-are-you-doing phone call once a month from a health worker to recovering heart attack patients helped boost their chance of survival by 50 percent over a group who got no such calls during the first year after their heart attacks.

And in a study of a group of breast cancer patients, the women who were able to talk most openly with other people about the stress of their illness had the best chance of recovery.

"The strain of not confiding emotional burdens of any kind creates a great physiological stress," says James Pennebaker, Ph.D., a psychologist at Southern Methodist University in Dallas. In his work, nonconfiders were found to have more health-related problems as well as more everyday ills than those who sought out someone to talk to.

So when the telephone company advertises, "Reach out and touch

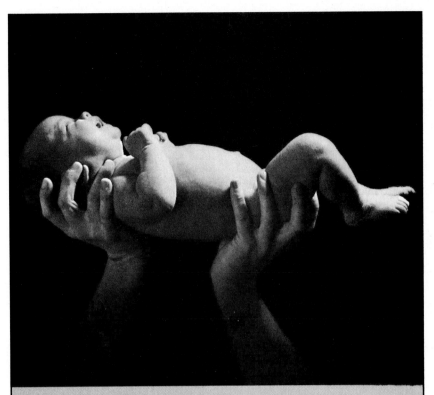

Breathe Like a Baby

Complete breathing using chest and abdomen (the way a baby does) can relax your body and calm and clear your mind, says veteran yoga teacher Ken Baxter of the Kripalu Center for Yoga and Health, Lenox, Massachusetts.

To learn to do it, lie on your back, with a pillow under your head. Draw your legs up, space your feet widely and lean your knees together. Lace your fingers loosely and rest your hands on your belly. Breathe deeply into your belly and feel your fingers gently separate. Fill your middle and upper chest, too. Let your shoulders relax. Next time you're in a tight spot, take 10 of these breaths and watch tension leave.

someone," they might well add, "and lower your stress."

LITTLE THINGS MEAN A LOT

"Put some gratitude in your attitude" is another suggestion for stress reduction from Kripalu's Dr. Dushkin.

Every night before he goes to sleep, no matter how grumpy he may be feeling, he makes himself count five things he's grateful for. It inevitably improves his mood and helps ensure a good night's sleep, he says.

"Be grateful for little things if you can't think of big ones," instructs Dr. Dushkin. "Be grateful when you find your shoes that they're in the same place you left them." (Anyone with a rowdy dog can appreciate that!)

Other handy tools for easing stress include a change in routine—a vacation, for instance—bearing in mind that your aim is to relax, not to get worked up over making every detail perfect or rushing to relax—

what one writer called "drag-racing to paradise."

A good book, a walk in the woods, a noncompetitive hobby, some time spent at the art museum, a pet to love and care for, a soothing sonata on the stereo, buying yourself a little present, a cup of hot peppermint tea with a dab of honey—these are easily available tools to break out of tension's grip. They are ways to persuade your mind that things aren't so bad after all—ways to turn off your brain's message to your body that it needs to be on guard.

And according to Dr. George Everly, one of the most effective tension relievers is the attitude embodied in the "Serenity Prayer"—

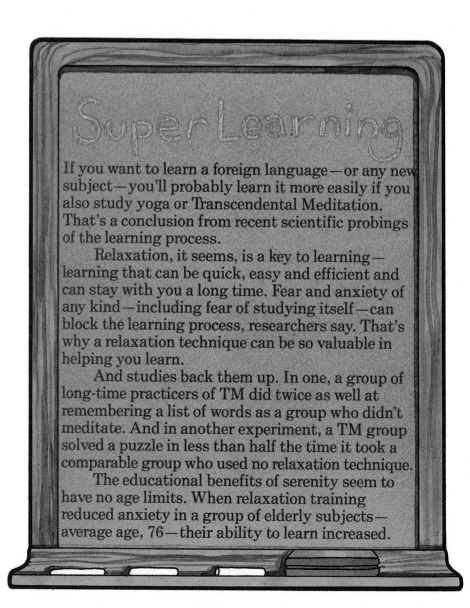

SuperLearning

If you want to learn a foreign language—or any new subject—you'll probably learn it more easily if you also study yoga or Transcendental Meditation. That's a conclusion from recent scientific probings of the learning process.

Relaxation, it seems, is a key to learning—learning that can be quick, easy and efficient and can stay with you a long time. Fear and anxiety of any kind—including fear of studying itself—can block the learning process, researchers say. That's why a relaxation technique can be so valuable in helping you learn.

And studies back them up. In one, a group of long-time practicers of TM did twice as well at remembering a list of words as a group who didn't meditate. And in another experiment, a TM group solved a puzzle in less than half the time it took a comparable group who used no relaxation technique.

The educational benefits of serenity seem to have no age limits. When relaxation training reduced anxiety in a group of elderly subjects—average age, 76—their ability to learn increased.

"God, grant me the serenity to accept the things I cannot change, the courage to change the things I can, and the wisdom to know the difference."

To know that difference sometimes takes a bit of introspection, say relaxation experts. Most of us have a need to take a periodic look at our values and the way we're treating ourselves—in short, at our attitudes, the slant we have on the world.

What do we tell ourselves when we make mistakes, as all humans do? Are our expectations of ourselves realistic? Or are we so demanding that we never allow ourselves to be pleased and proud of ourselves?

Do we keep rushing just to avoid those moments when we might have to look at ourselves and ask, "Where am I headed and how am I getting there? Is this really how I want to be living my life?"

These self-examinations (many people find a pencil and paper come in handy and a diary gives even more perspective) help us find the base inside ourselves that is the true source of peace—being in touch with our own needs and feelings rather than simply reacting to external pressures.

Self-examination can foster the kinds of attitudes that recent studies have shown to be helpful in handling stressful situations. A feeling of control, for instance—the knowledge that you are not powerless, that you can influence your fate. A sense of being committed, also—believing in what you are doing. And finally, the gift of seeing the positive side of difficult situations—that they are opportunities to learn and grow. Indeed, a recent psychological survey has shown that people who have successfully passed through extremely stressful life events (such as a personal tragedy) can be psychologically healthier than those of us who haven't been through really trying times.

And if you have difficulty scouting your own interior, you might consider help from a therapist or anyone who can assist you in examining the terrain of your own attitudes. Remember—and here's a good attitude to start with—that reaching for help is a sign of strength, not weakness.

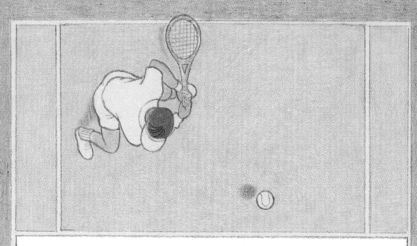

How to Play the Inner Game

Flow. That's the word athletes use when moves, timing and mental attitude come together with effortless grace in a winning performance.

The funny thing is, the athletes say, they had often imagined just such a performance over and over in their minds.

It's not surprising, say psychologists. For years they have recommended that same method for improving sports performance. And whether your game is rugby or marbles,

mentally playing what's been called the inner game can improve your skill.

How does it work? When you're in a deeply relaxed state and visualize yourself performing, say researchers, your mind and muscles stage a minirehearsal for the real thing. (The extra electrical output of your muscles is actually measurable.)

Though fantasizing can't replace training, it can be a valuable adjunct, say experts.

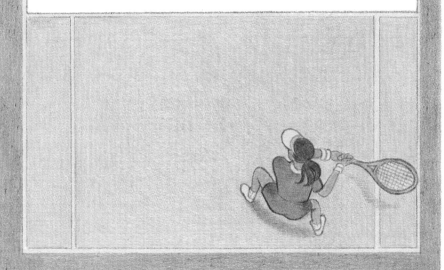

Water Therapy

Perhaps it's because we *are* mostly water, each cell like a tiny pool. Or because we spent the first months of existence buoyed in a warm capsule of liquid. Or because the source of all life is probably the ocean, and a genetic message pulls us back to water like the moon pulls the tide. But whatever the reason, water soothes and restores us; it literally washes away worries and cares. Before you soak, however, consult your doctor if you are pregnant or have a chronic or serious health problem.

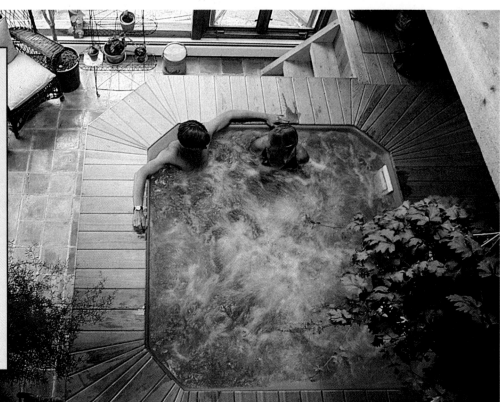

Getting Tubby

It's not just for Californians anymore. The hot tub's appeal has spread nationwide. Along with the more modestly sized Jacuzzis and whirlpools, these tubs offer pulsing jets of water that massage as well as warm for muscular healing and calming benefits.

Foot Bath

"Go soak your feet" may be just plain good advice for someone with a tension headache. The warm (less than 100°F), wet heat on your lower extremities sends a signal to relax to the constricted, pain-producing veins and muscles in your head, say experts.

A Shower Massage—and More

The spray of a hot shower beating on the back of a sore neck. Ah-h-h—it feels so good! But a shower can do more than relax sore muscles; it can energize you, too. When you're weary but need to keep going, alternate a few minutes of really hot water with as cold a splash as you can stand. Repeat 3 to 5 times, always ending with cold, for sheer exhilaration.

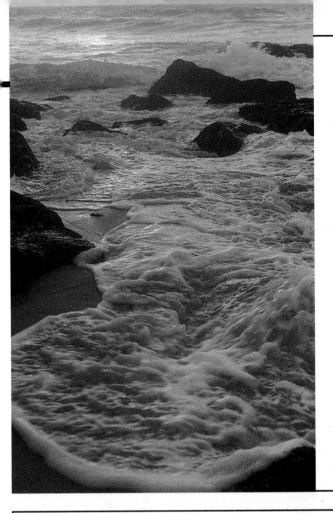

The Serenity of the Sea

You can almost feel it now . . . the warmth of the sun wrapping you like a cocoon, the sound of the surf soothing your thoughts and mellowing your mood. Surf sounds are so-o-o-o soothing they're even featured on many relaxation tapes. When you're on the beach, you get not only the rhythmic pounding of the waves but also those shoreline, good-mood, negative ions.

Saunas and Steam Baths

Curiously refreshing. No, not Schweppes. We're talking saunas and steam baths. Researchers have tried for decades to scientifically explain the appeal of sitting in a hot box and working up a sweat. One medical wag speculated that people enjoy saunas and steam baths because it feels so good to get out! Well, no one knows why they make you feel good, but they do. However, their effect depends on the individual. Some say they relax; some say they energize. But the bottom line on saunas and steam baths is that people simply love them.

The Bath: A Whole-Body Healer

Soaking in a lukewarm bath sends a telegram to your brain that says "relax." A hotter bath can ease sore muscles. But be forewarned. Soak in a really hot tub for 30 minutes or longer and you may wind up so limp you'll fall asleep.

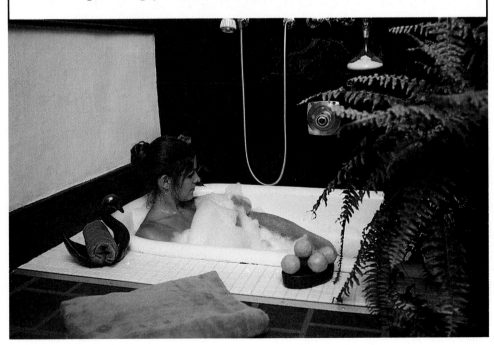

9

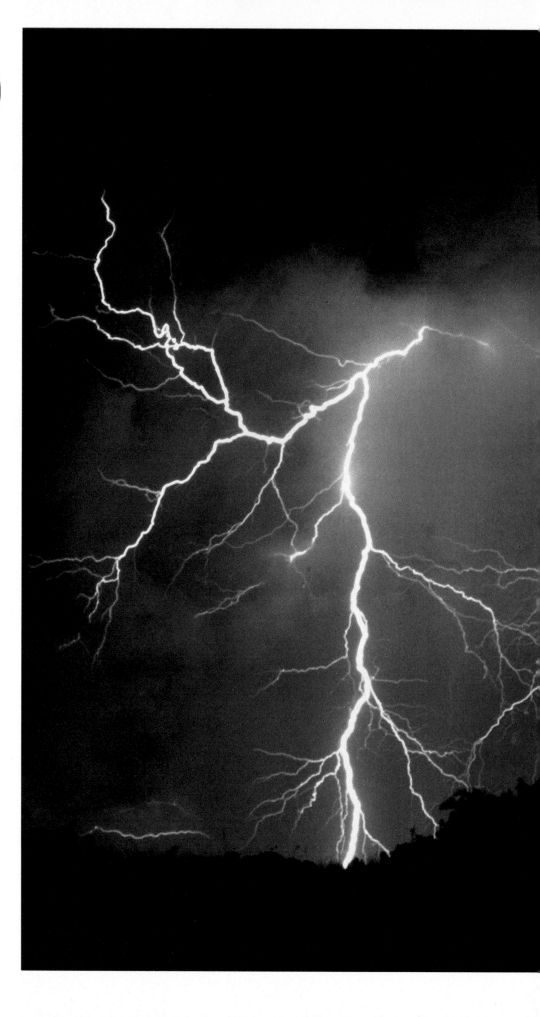

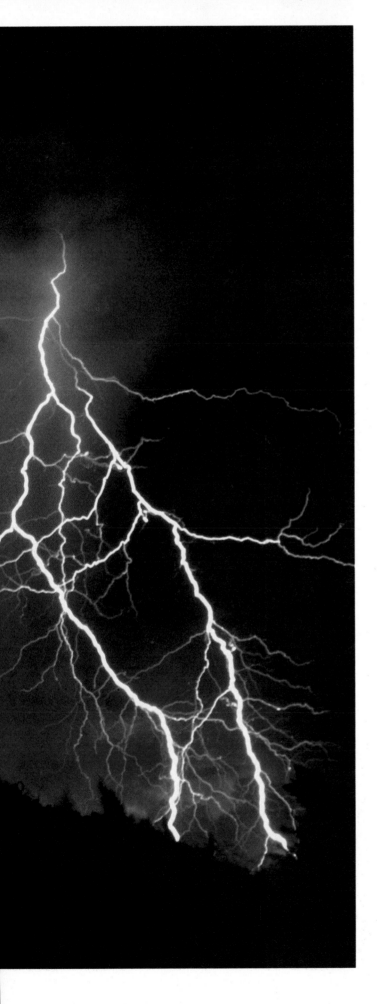

Energy and the Environment

The people, places and things that surround us can have a powerful impact on our vitality.

Are you concerned about the environment? No, we're not talking about the toxic waste dump that wants to move next door or about having to clean a couple of tons of crude diesel oil off several miles of beach. We're talking about your *personal* environment—all those little taken-for-granted things that go together to make up the space around you.

Stop and think for a second. Look outside. What's the weather like? Is it warm and muggy or chilly and dry? What about the light? Are you sitting in front of an open window or basking in the glow of fluorescent tubing? Is it noisy or quiet? What colors surround you? Is your chair comfortable? How about your friends and co-workers—what kind of people are they, nasty or nice? These are things we mostly don't think about in terms of personal energy. But they have an effect on us, whether we know it or not.

One doctor and weather expert, for example, says that when clouds roll in and the temperature drops, a bad night's sleep may be part of the forecast. And studies show that some people who live in noisy neighborhoods (like under the landing paths of a major airport) have a tough time feeling refreshed and relaxed—even their blood pressure is uptight. Yet these people might never connect their insomnia or tension with the environmental factor.

And that's a shame, since discovering the black hole that's sucking your energy is the first step toward plugging it up. Which is what this chapter is all about—discovering. Light. Color. Weather. Sound. And all the other things in the world around you that can energize—or enervate—the world within.

Weather

Noted sex researcher Alfred Kinsey once noted that the only true aphrodisiacs were exercise, fresh air, sunshine, good food and enough sleep. Obviously, the right weather can give you two out of five.

But if fresh air and sunshine can turn you on, what happens when the skies are gray and the air gets so muggy that you feel like you could grab a handful and wring out a quart of water?

According to Stephen Rosen, Ph.D., director of the Weather Sensitivity Research Center in New York City, for those individuals who are "weather sensitive," these changes can have a strong effect on their energy level and their health, as well. Specifically he has observed that:

- What some would call "extremely good weather"—characterized by a hot, dry wind—makes people feel less healthy in general, reduces their desire to work and actually decreases their work output. There's also a greater chance of them being involved in a household or automobile accident, probably because they aren't concentrating very well.

- When a change in the weather is just around the corner, people tend not to feel well—or not to feel much like working. They may become more sensitive to pain and again are more at risk of having an accident.

- When the temperature and humidity are both high, it's no surpirse that the warm, moist weather makes many people feel tired; it also may disturb their sleep and increase their chance of having an accident.

- Finally, when cool, dry air arrives (the kind that pushes the barometer up to the high numbers), spirits are boosted and people feel more lively. Their reaction time may be a bit slower, however, and there is some reason to believe that they may actually need more sleep—especially if the weather has been heading in this direction for some time.

It's important to remember that these observations are mostly true for people who are *weather sensitive:* those who feel a real change in their health and attitude when there's a change in the weather.

Who are these people whose moods and energy levels shift with the wind? One-third to two-thirds of the population, say weather researchers. But it isn't an across-the-board percentage.

Tiredness, bad moods and disinclination to work are the most frequent complaints of weather-sensitive people, says Dr. Rosen. And out of the three, tiredness is the most pronounced single complaint.

GETTING ALONG WITH THE WEATHER

This doesn't mean, however, that people who are sensitive to the weather are doomed to a life of fluctuating weariness.

There *are* things you can do to lessen sensitivity and reclaim some of the energy that bad weather drains away.

Edgar Folk, Ph.D., a professor of physiology at the University of Iowa, explains that "people vary a great deal" in their ability to adapt to the weather. Some of those variables, like age and ancestry, are beyond our control. But knowing that people who exercise regularly can tolerate weather changes better than their sedentary companions may give you another incentive to get started on that workout program you keep putting off.

Dr. Folk also points out that almost everyone—even those who don't consider themselves weather sensitive—suffers a distinct loss of vitality when exposed to excessive heat or cold. He feels that the problem is a question of adjustment— that people don't allow themselves time to get accustomed to these extremes of temperature. We can temper their effects, he says, by a process called acclimatization.

If it suddenly becomes very cold, for instance, you should begin to acclimatize yourself with a relatively brief exposure to the weather outdoors to begin with, then gradually

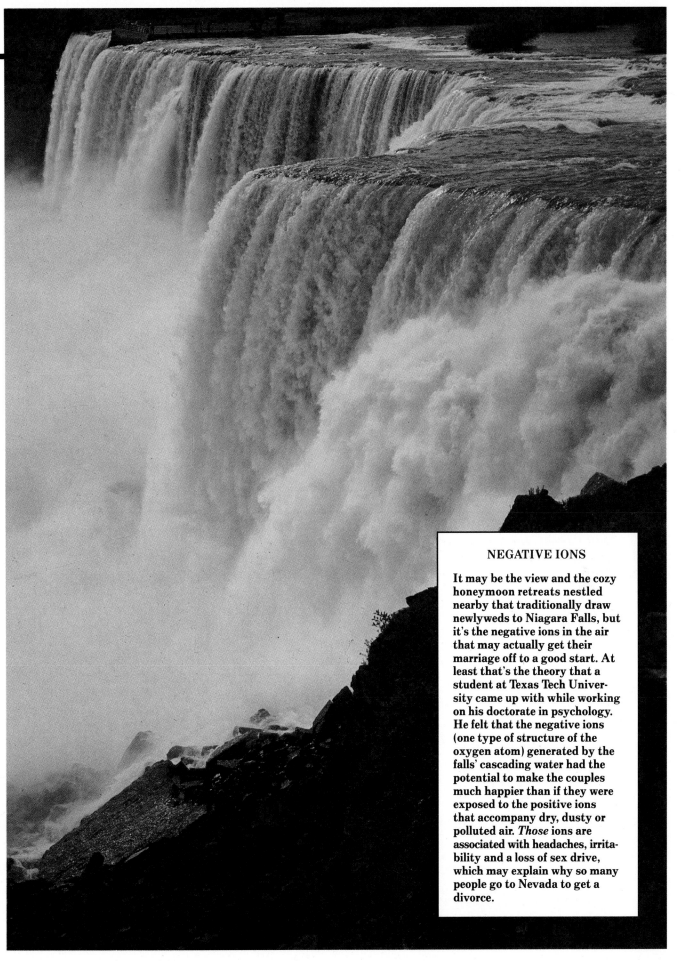

NEGATIVE IONS

It may be the view and the cozy honeymoon retreats nestled nearby that traditionally draw newlyweds to Niagara Falls, but it's the negative ions in the air that may actually get their marriage off to a good start. At least that's the theory that a student at Texas Tech University came up with while working on his doctorate in psychology. He felt that the negative ions (one type of structure of the oxygen atom) generated by the falls' cascading water had the potential to make the couples much happier than if they were exposed to the positive ions that accompany dry, dusty or polluted air. *Those* ions are associated with headaches, irritability and a loss of sex drive, which may explain why so many people go to Nevada to get a divorce.

increase your time and activities outside a little bit more each day. After a week to ten days of this gradual exposure, you'll be much better prepared to handle a lot of time outside on a real deep-freeze of a day.

The process works the same when the weather suddenly turns hot. Essentially, you want to avoid sending your body into a kind of climatic shock by exposing yourself to too much, too soon. "If you work your way into the weather," Dr. Folk explains, "you can moderate the effect it has on you."

But don't feel that the arrival of winter naturally means a drop in your energy levels along with the temperature. "Man actually has a higher metabolism in the winter to compensate for the colder weather," explains Dr. Folk. As an example, he notes that "in the winter you don't walk slowly between buildings. You

hurry, and you tend to keep hurrying once you're inside."

If that scenario doesn't describe you, then you should try taking some time to acclimatize yourself the next time a cold spell hits hard. If your body is properly prepared, cold weather should boost your energy levels.

Acclimatization becomes especially important, however, when newspapers run pictures of fried eggs sizzling on the sidewalk. "There's no doubt that heat is debilitating," says Dr. Folk. "You're naturally going to have more energy if you're comfortable and cool."

You can guard your energy valuables against thieving heat by paying attention—a constant excessive rise in body temperature while you're exercising or any excessive rise while you're sedentary is a signal of oncoming heat fatigue and possible exhaustion. Again, acclimatizing your-

Your Energy Highs and Lows

The changes in the weather that make the mercury in a barometer go up and down can have the same effect on your energy level. Slow, gradual changes in the barometric pressure don't cause drastic

changes in energy. But rapid changes are strong enough to be felt inside buildings and have a distinct effect on almost everyone, even those who aren't considered weather sensitive.

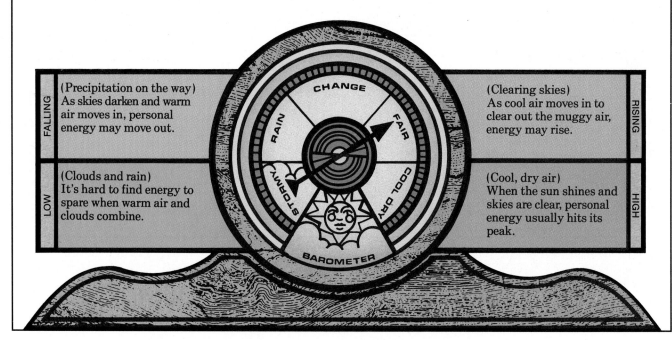

FALLING

(Precipitation on the way) As skies darken and warm air moves in, personal energy may move out.

LOW

(Clouds and rain) It's hard to find energy to spare when warm air and clouds combine.

RISING

(Clearing skies) As cool air moves in to clear out the muggy air, energy may rise.

HIGH

(Cool, dry air) When the sun shines and skies are clear, personal energy usually hits its peak.

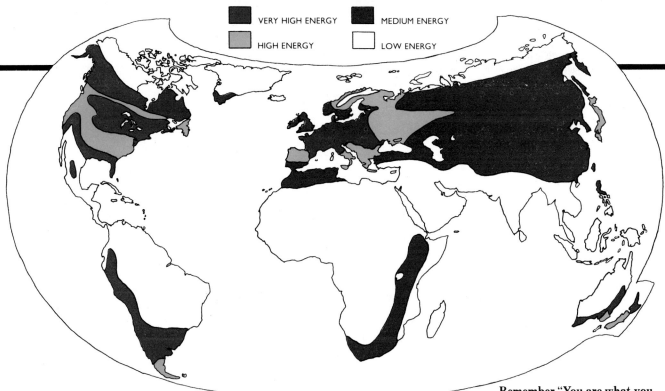

VERY HIGH ENERGY MEDIUM ENERGY

HIGH ENERGY LOW ENERGY

self can help you to tolerate the heat better, but if your temperature is climbing along with the thermometer, take steps to protect yourself.

"If the humidity is not too high," explains Dr. Folk, "water will help. It doesn't even have to be especially cold—just wash your hands and face. But if the humidity is high, water alone doesn't help—you have to get cooler." If air conditioning or a much cooler area isn't immediately available, Dr. Folk suggests a cool bath or shower. "You can't overemphasize humidity," he says.

And that's when you pray for a nice breeze, right? After all, everyone knows that the effect of a stiff breeze will be to cool you off on a hot summer day.

"Mostly that's true," Dr. Folk says. "Generally a breeze will refresh you when it's hot. If the temperature is 85°, for instance, a 20-mile-per-hour wind will make it feel more like 82°."

When it's really hot, however, that breeze will work *against* you. It's called the Driscoll breeze factor—a recent discovery that shows there is actually a reversal of the breeze effect when the temperature hits between 90° and 95°F, just when we seek breezy relief the most. "If the temperature is 95°, that same 20-mile-per-hour wind will now make it seem like it's 97°," he says. "You're actually *gaining* heat from the breeze."

So remember to take the same

cool-down precautions—drinking plenty of water; taking cool baths or showers; eating foods rich in potassium (which is lost in perspiration), like watermelons and bananas; wearing loose fabrics that "breathe," like cotton; and exercising in the cool of the day.

WHEN NEGATIVE IS POSITIVE

Another way a hot wind may rob you of energy is by creating an excess of positive ions in the air. Ions are created when electrons either detach from or hook onto oxygen molecules in the air. And the *positive* ions generated by a hot, dry wind—like the legendary "witches' winds" of the world, the sirocco in Italy (also called the father of depression), France's mistral, Austria's foehn, the chinook that comes down out of the Rockies and the Santa Ana that blows into California from the desert— are generally associated with negative effects on human beings: moodiness, headaches, fatigue. The *negative* ions that are found around cascading water (like waterfalls or oceans) are thought to make people feel positive— happier and more energetic.

But you don't need to go to the beach or a waterfall to raise your spirits. Just take a shower. The action of the cascading water will generate negative ions all around you.

Remember "You are what you eat"? Maybe that should be changed to "You are where you live," since some researchers feel that different areas of the globe seem to endow their residents with significantly different levels of energy. The magic zone bursting with great cities and cultural achievements seem to be located in a narrow band running between 30° and 60° north latitude—an area of bracing but moderate temperatures with strong seasonal changes. Cities such as New York, Chicago, Los Angeles, London, Paris, Rome and Tokyo are all located here. Yale geographer Ellsworth Huntington, who did the study back in the 1930s, defused possible charges of racism by observing that farmers in the northern U.S., both black and white, consistently worked more to improve their land than either black or white Southern farmers. It is the northern climate, he feels, that gives those farmers more "vigor."

Pollution

When it comes to energy and health, most pollution seems like a kind of environmental rash—vaguely uncomfortable and unsightly, but not too bothersome. But pollution can actually rob you of energy, even *permanently*. That's what it did to 63 people in Belgium, 19 in Pittsburgh and 4,000 in London— all victims of supertoxic smogs that blanketed those areas like a filthy shroud. That's the worst it gets, of course. But it's not always much better. Take lead, for instance.

Parents know not to let their children eat paint chips because of the possibility of lead poisoning, yet the air we breathe every day contains lead, mostly from car exhaust.

"Health problems caused by exposure to low levels of lead are common," explains Herbert Needleman, M.D., an expert on lead poisoning, adding that many physicians may not relate the initial symptoms of fatigue, irritability and depression to the toxic pollutant.

Luckily, there is a way to combat this nasty substance. Researchers at the Brain Bio Center in Princeton, New Jersey, found that high intakes of vitamin C and zinc not only caused levels of lead in the blood of the study participants to diminish, but also may have "flushed" lead already present out of their bodies. Their conclusion was that "by increasing zinc and vitamin C intake, everyone could be better protected against the inevitable lead exposure that is part of modern life."

ROAD POLLUTION— EVERYONE'S PROBLEM

Hopefully, lead in the air will become less of a problem as leaded gasoline is slowly phased out. But that won't make the ozone situation any better. The U.S. Department of Transportation studied the effects of air pollution on cyclists who biked to work in Washington, D.C., and found that more than one-third of the cyclists were breathing levels of ozone that exceeded national standards.

Besides ozone, the cyclists were exposed to carbon monoxide from car exhausts in quantities high enough to be easily detected in their blood. The result was fatigue—directly related to the toxic gases inhaled on the route. And it was even worse for drivers on four wheels— those inside cars had much higher levels of carbon monoxide in their blood than the cyclists, apparently from being trapped in rush hour traffic.

So what can you do, short of quitting your job? Some scientists think you might want to increase your stores of vitamin E.

An antioxidant, vitamin E has been found to protect against the ozone that threatens to drain our energy and damage our lungs. Daniel B. Menzel, Ph.D., director of the laboratory of environmental pharmacology and toxicology at Duke University Medical Center, suggests that 200 international units (I.U.) of vitamin E "should help protect the body against the stress of air pollution." Vitamin E also helps zinc and vitamin C to work against the unwelcome lead in your system.

The pollution threat isn't just an occasional event limited to specific, obvious areas. "Air pollution is not confined to metropolitan areas," says Dr. Menzel. "The amount of ozone in certain rural areas of New Jersey is greater than in downtown Manhattan."

SELENIUM AND ALLERGIC FATIGUE

You know how you feel when you have the flu: head throbbing, muscles aching—a real energy-zapping experience. You're too weak to even lift your head off the pillow.

Following overexposure to carbon monoxide on a research project, Steven A. Levine, Ph.D., developed flulike symptoms that persisted for years. After numerous attempts to find out what was wrong with him, Dr. Levine realized that he was reacting to the chemical products in the modern world around him. He was literally allergic to the environment. For years he sought a solution, but nothing seemed to work. Then he heard about the protective qualities

Indoor Air Pollution

One of the reasons that indoor pollution may be more serious than the stuff out-of-doors is that we spend about 80 percent of our time inside, and new, efficient, heavily insulated houses have the potential to trap a lot of stale air and contaminants that literally used to blow out the window. The house may retain *its* energy, but the inhabitants can lose much of theirs.

Fatigue, tiredness, inability to concentrate, lethargy, light-headedness, weakness, a run-down feeling, morning dizziness and depression—all were the initial allergic reactions of people whose problems were later traced to simply living in their own homes.

Alfred V. Zamm, M.D., author of the book *Why Your House May Endanger Your Health*, cites a number of dangerous vapors that are present—and trapped—in most modern homes. He uses the broad term "mental dysfunction" to describe the many and varied symptoms, including chronic tiredness, that they can cause in susceptible persons. ("Susceptible" is important because it applies to only a small percentage of the population.) One cure is to have people with these problems remove as many of the offending sources of pollution as they can until their symptoms disappear.

Adequate ventilation is one of the best defenses against feeling like your house fell on you. No one knows for sure just how much fresh air will dilute indoor pollutants to a safe level, but an accepted standard is that *all* the stale air in a home should be exchanged for fresh air every 2 to 3 hours.

of the trace mineral selenium, and he began treating himself. Almost like a miracle, his symptoms disappeared. When he stopped the selenium, the flulike symptoms reappeared. So he went back to the selenium and the symptoms went away again.

Of course, few people react as strongly to their environment as Dr. Levine. But some experts believe that anyone living in polluted areas—large cities, areas surrounding industry, or high-traffic areas—will suffer to some degree from ecological illness and be unaware of it. They may

simply feel tired all the time. Protection with selenium may help fight this kind of fatigue.

Working with Michael Rosenbaum, M.D., of Mill Valley, California, Dr. Levine found that selenium supplements significantly improved half of their patients suffering from ecological illness. However, selenium should always be taken with caution. Selenium at high doses can be toxic. That's why you should take this mineral under the supervision of a doctor, and never take more than 200 micrograms a day.

Allergic Hazards

A. Gas stove— One small study showed that after only 1 hour, a gas stove can produce enough toxic gases to rival L.A. smog.

B. Gas heat— Some heaters may pollute the air to a level 3 times higher than federal standards.

C. Insulation and wallboard—If formaldehyde is an ingredient in these materials, it can seep out.

D. Under the sink—Cleaning aids can contain toxic chemicals.

E. The bathroom— Hair sprays, colognes, air fresheners, nail polish and deodorants can cause reactions.

F. The garage—If it's attached to the house, exhaust and oil fumes can seep inside.

G. The basement— Paints and other workbench hazards, mold and mildew can cause problems.

The People Around Us

Relationships are directly related to your energy level, says Charles T. Kuntzleman, Ed.D., author of *Maximum Personal Energy*. A "dynamic, positive relationship with another human being is just the ticket for an energetic life."

"On the other hand," he admits, "negative relationships produce a sense of turmoil that merely adds to the problems that you already have." Dealing with negative people, he says, leaves you "little energy left over to function as a normal member of society . . . the bounce leaves

your step, fatigue sets in earlier."

Gordon M. Hart, Ph.D., a counseling psychologist at Philadelphia's Temple University, explains how people should choose their friends for maximum energy.

"We use people around us as energizers, to get us up and motivate us—people whom we like, people who give us smiles, who listen to us," he says. "It's a matter of trying to seek out these people in a real conscious way, and I don't think that a lot of people know how to do that."

Dr. Hart feels that most of us

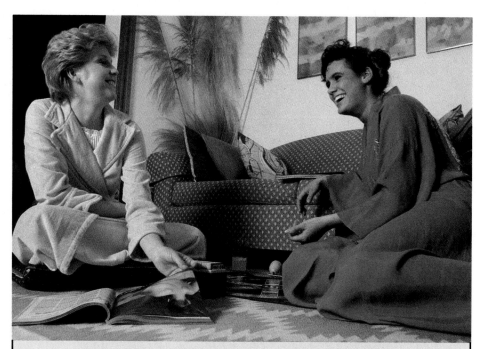

Finding the Perfect Roommate

When it comes to finding a compatible roommate, "It's a matter of finding somebody similar enough to you but not alike; dissimilar from you but not totally opposite," says Gordon M. Hart, Ph.D., counseling psychologist at Temple University.

He suggests rating them (and yourself) on a scale of 1 (no energy) to 10 (high energy).

If you're a 4, you can handle a wide range of people, but your ideal roommate would be a 6. If you're a 9, then you could well stand someone at the 3 or 4 level, since no one would ever want to live next door to two 9s. The potential racket that two high-energy people can create could be unbearable. If you're a 1 or a 2, you should look for a 7 or an 8.

aren't very good judges of character.

"We have a sort of innate sense," he explains, "but talking with other people—friends, relatives, professionals—can help us home in on what we really like about other people—and about ourselves. If we want to be more energetic, we're going to have to put up some barriers to keep away the people who are likely to drain us."

But how do we get energy givers into our lives while leaving the energy robbers behind?

"What I suggest is that someone should actually make a list of the people in their environment, including at work, and then make a list of people who they feel would be more positive for them. It could be people they know in a peripheral sort of way—that they met at a party or see on the bus. And then decide whether or not they want to reach out to some new people and kind of put the brakes on their relationship with some others. That can be done in a real pen-and-pencil sort of way."

If you need help doing this exercise, Dr. Hart feels you should approach a friend whom you trust and who has some of the same people in common "so that you can get a kind of second opinion."

Dr. Hart makes it clear that those making a list need to take a hard look at what kind of energy *they* give off as well. You can attract energetic people much more easily when you yourself are an energetic person. Do you eat properly? Are you physically active? These are good questions to ask yourself to measure your own energy level.

Dr. Hart feels that people who work at keeping in shape make better friends and are better people to be around because of their sense of psychological well-being. "It helps you to be the kind of person that is easiest to get along with," he explains, "a person who is more likely to be sensitive to the needs of others, whether that means being an energizer or a calmer.

"People who feel better about themselves make the best friends and have the most energy to give—and that's what you're looking for." In short, energy attracts energy.

The Energy Vampires

Every morning they rise in search of victims, following the scent of fresh, energetic blood to its source and then, creeping up from behind, they strike with the dreaded words, "Oh, you're not busy, are you?" The energy vampire has struck again, draining his helpless co-worker with endless, boring stories of home, family, this week's illness and last night's television. How can you protect yourself? A fierce counter-attack with garlic and a crucifix before the baby pictures come out? A wooden stake?

No (thank God)! A study commissioned by GF Business Equipment, Inc., of Youngstown, Ohio, suggests that some less drastic tactics may be equally effective.

- Arrange your office furniture so that you don't face the center of activity. People are less likely to visit if your back is to them.
- Be direct. Simply say that you're sorry, but you can't be disturbed right now. If you don't want to appear antisocial, go out of your way to be nice to these people at other times.
- Keep your responses brief; your tone of voice can convey your lack of interest.
- Don't look into the eyes of the vampire. It's hard for them to keep up a conversation without your eye contact.
- Keep your pen or pencil poised; don't take your fingers off the keyboard. They're hints you want to get back to work.
- Keep the phone in your hand or pick it up; make it clear that you need to make a call.
- Stand up when you want your visitor to leave. Almost everyone gets this message.
- Shuffle papers, make notes. It should be obvious that you want to get back to work.

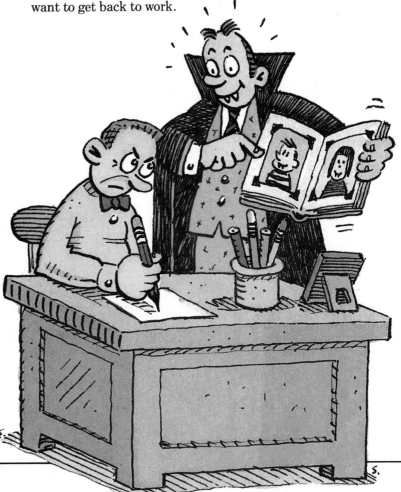

Noise

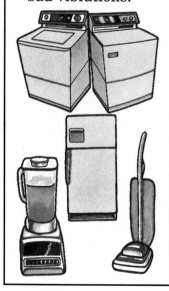
"**N**oise" means *any* unwanted sound, but especially the loud and objectionable variety: Kids carrying those "boom box" radios with massive crackling speakers spewing out just the kind of music you never wanted to hear. An airplane committing sonic flatulence in the sky overhead. A motorcycle desperately in need of a muffler. As we know all too well, the list is neverending. And always annoying.

Londoners were asked the question, "If you could change just one of the things you don't like about living here, which would you choose?" They decided they could live with the slums, the dirt and the smoke—if only something could be done about the noise!

The single most obvious way that noise can rob our energy is very direct—it can keep us from falling asleep or wake us up after we finally get there. "It is an undisputed fact that adequate sleep is a physiological necessity," explains William Burns, author of *Noise and Man*.

Burns confirms a suspicion that many of us have held: Some people literally can "sleep through anything." They seem to have the ability to become accustomed to almost any level or type of noise. The rest of us, however, are likely to suffer the occasional rude awakening—especially from intermittent sounds like airplane and traffic noise.

One possible way to shield yourself from the noisy world at night is to strike back with white noise. Sheldon Cohen, Ph.D., a professor of psychology at Carnegie-Mellon University in Pittsburgh, suggests "masking" the unwanted sounds with your own continuous background noise.

A special machine that generates a constant, soothing background sound would be the best bet, but Dr. Cohen says that the hum of a fan or an air conditioner can also be very effective. He says no to a radio, however. Even turned down very low, it would still be conveying too much real information to be an unintrusive backdrop.

On nights when the diesel trucks do a dance outside your window every hour, white noise may lose out to black blares, blasts, booms and bangs. When that happens, your energy levels the next day are going to be down, but only for the first 2 hours of the day. So don't try to set the world on fire in the morning. You'll do better later on.

This differs from actual *sleep deprivation*, which causes performance to slide much later in the day. So, if you didn't sleep at all, you might want to try to leave work early, after accomplishing as much as you can.

RACKET IN THE WORKPLACE

A noisy place of business doesn't seem to affect the pace of employees as much as it affects their accuracy. People exposed to noise—*especially* those who are trying to do a good job—make more mistakes. But in surveys, less than half of those interviewed felt that work noise disturbed them.

Cotton weavers, for instance, were certain that noise wasn't affecting their performance. Yet, when they were asked to wear earplugs, their work efficiency improved. Even though they didn't like wearing the plugs, their work efficiency improved signifcantly.

Continuous noise is a hidden enemy. Like the cotton weavers, we don't notice the effect, but it steadily decreases our reaction time. That's a sure sign of sagging energy levels.

High levels of noise act more directly. Massive auditory stimulation leads to persistent reports of excessive fatigue, nausea and disorientation.

The Environmental Protection Agency notes that one of the most common effects of noise exposure is exhaustion. Leonard Woodcock, former president of the United Auto Workers, noticed that some of the members of his union "find themselves unusually fatigued at the end of the day compared to their fellow workers who are not exposed to much noise."

The best advice to avoid coming home from work all noised-out is to wear ear protectors on the job. A researcher in Copenhagen who is working on the harmful psychological effects of noise thinks that companies should provide a wide variety of ear protectors for workers to choose from.

If your place of employment isn't responsive in this area, take the initiative and check out sporting goods stores. They feature a wide variety of types and styles of ear protectors for gun fanciers. Remember, you want something that will be comfortable over a long shift.

There is little doubt that noise robs energy. Tiredness and fatigue are the most common physical complaints of people exposed to noise. It can also strike our minds.

Teachers exposed to excessive noise in the classroom felt that it made them—and their students—more tired and less inclined to work. The proof showed up in a study: When faced with complex puzzles, children who attended schools in noisy areas gave up faster than children in quieter schools.

So noise attacks us at home, at work, at school and everywhere in between. What can we do to keep its loud fingers out of our energy pocket?

Some sounds can be controlled. Talk to neighbors about noisy pets, stereos, TVs and mufflers that don't muffle anymore. Do a little sound-proofing at home and in the car.

You can also change your mind. Annoyance, a prime factor in raising the blood pressure and draining your energy, may largely be a matter of personal perception.

Residents living near a Swedish air force base complained less about the noise after they received a souvenir book commemorating the base's 50th anniversary. The book suggested that local residents were proud to live near a base so important to their national security. Residents who didn't get the book continued to complain.

So, one person's noise can be another's music. For example, explains Dr. Cohen, the noise of a factory working at peak performance is a sweet sound to the factory owner, but it can be really irritating to the family living next door.

Music Is the Magic That Keeps You Movin'

After a long day's work that began and ended with a grueling commute, Kathy was beyond mere exhaustion. "I was standing at the sink," she remembers, "just staring into space with no energy to even *think* about getting dinner together." Then a Bruce Springsteen song came on the radio. "It was a real rocker," she says, "and suddenly I was moving my feet—almost dancing! I turned the music up and dinner became a breeze instead of a chore. *And* I met my husband at the door with a big smile instead of him finding me collapsed in a chair!"

Kathy's story is far from unique. At the famed Aerobics Center of Kenneth Cooper, M.D., in Dallas, 18-year-old Blake Boyd listened to tapes while running on a high-speed treadmill. He lasted over 32 minutes—beating the previous record that had been set by a marathon runner—and gave the credit to Michael Jackson. "The music helped pass the time and get my mind off how much my legs hurt," explained Boyd.

When Ohio State University scientist Eric Miller tested joggers, they reported that their exercise felt easier when accompanied by music. More important, Miller found that those who listened while they worked out actually had lower levels of endorphins—morphinelike chemicals produced by the brain in times of stress.

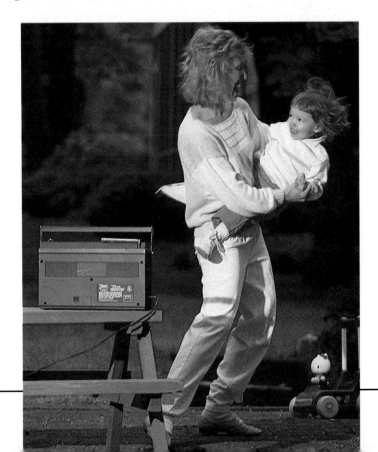

Light

When officials at the Burnett Park Zoo in Syracuse, New York, installed floodlights as a defense against vandalism, they ended up with more than a simple reduction in graffiti and broken glass.

The zoo "had been turned into a veritable maternity ward," noted one onlooker. The cougars produced a new litter, the geese laid eggs, 8 new lambs and 20 young deer were born—and a bear cub, a baby wallabee and a young chimpanzee were soon added to the population.

At the Houston Zoological Gardens, Jozef Laszlo wondered if a lack of sunlight was contributing to the premature deaths of many snakes and lizards. He installed special full-spectrum fluorescent lights that mimicked true sunlight and soon noted that the creatures became more healthy and active.

These energizing effects aren't limited to animals, and zookeepers aren't the only ones who realize it. In Norway, for instance, every employee must be exposed to a certain amount of natural lighting. It's the *law*.

And in Russia, one group of researchers found that individuals who received extra doses of ultraviolet light had better reaction times, less eye fatigue and a greater capacity for work than those who didn't get the extra ultraviolet. Full-spectrum light also was found to increase the body's resistance to environmental pollutants—and it significantly improved the working capacity and academic performance of school children. Such lighting is now mandated in many indoor environments in the USSR.

And there's more. Studies in the 1940s determined that in the workplace, the *quality* of the light is just as important as the quantity. The right kinds of light can improve the way people feel, while the wrong kinds can have a negative effect on their health and performance. Fatigue is a direct result of lackluster lighting.

Workers themselves will back this up. In a European survey, employees stated that good lighting was more important than good ventilation, a comfortable temperature or even enough space to work. In the United States, a Louis Harris poll found that "good lighting was . . . the most important factor affecting personal comfort on the job."

In short, there seems to be a basic human requirement—as essential as the one for vitamins—for light. And not just any light.

"If man is to be confined for long hours, kept out of nature and away from the sun, he will need balanced light that emits a fairly full spectrum, including some ultraviolet," says Faber Birren in his book *Color and Human Response.*

SADness and the Midnight Sun

A travel article on the wonders of Iceland leads off by mentioning that Icelanders "are some of the best partiers in the world" and that the best time to observe such behavior is in the summer "when daylight may last 24 hours."

So what happens to these fun lovers in the winter, when the sun doesn't show its face for what seems like forever? They develop Seasonal Affective Disorder; like its initials, it makes them SAD. The syndrome is characterized by depression, fatigue, sleepiness and weight gain.

Medical specialists in the relatively new field of phototherapy have found that they can cure the depression and raise the energy levels of these SAD patients by exposing them to high levels of the kind of full-spectrum light that mimics the sun. They try to fool the patients' brains into thinking it's really summer.

That's what Alfred Lewy, M.D., Ph.D., did to chase the blues away from a patient whose moods had previously been brightened only by the onset of spring. To give him "spring days in the winter," Dr. Lewy extended the patient's "day" by 3 hours in the morning and 3 hours in the afternoon by using high levels of light. After a few days the depression lifted.

So be generous with your light in the winter if you feel a little draggy. Dr. Lewy recommends you get outdoors early in the day, preferably as soon as the sun comes up.

SEEKING SOLAR ENERGY

But what does "full spectrum" mean? What's so special about ultraviolet?

The solar rays that beam down on us as sunshine contain this mysterious ultraviolet light. The "middle range" of this light is what gives us a healthy-looking tan—or a lobsterlike burn. The "far end" of the scale is more harmful, but not much of it gets through the ozone layer that surrounds the earth. The "low end" of the scale—the "near ultraviolet" rays—is the part we can't live without. And we can't get it from normal indoor lights.

Regular incandescent light bulbs provide almost no ultraviolet light, and regular fluorescents seem to actually *absorb* it—constituting a double threat by competing with humans for what little may be around.

There's only one genuine source for the real thing—the sun.

Dr. Edgar Folk of the University of Iowa explains that exposure to the sun does much more than just bronze bodies and manufacture vitamin D.

Because it actually is radiation, sunlight doesn't stop at the surface—it penetrates the hair and skull to get where it has to go. That sunlight gets in and activates one of the most important glands in the head, the pineal gland, to produce a profound effect on our energy level, says Dr. Folk. "It doesn't make us hyperactive, but there's a feeling of more energy and more willingness to use it." He calls a healthy, functioning pineal gland, "the pathway to energy." When it's working properly, more hours of daylight mean more hours of activity.

In fact, Dr. Folk feels that it is generally accepted that the effects of "cabin fever" in the North during the cold winters are at least partially due to the lack of stimulating sunlight. He should know—he has some personal experience with the opposite sensation.

"I spent some time in the Arctic, working during the season of continuous daylight there, and it really drives you to do more. You almost resent having to go to sleep," he says.

So it seems that a summer spent in the Arctic may be the ultimate in energizing vacations. But what about closer to home?

BARELY HEALTHY

"We were born naked," reminds John M. Douglass, M.D., a Los Angeles specialist in internal medicine and health improvement. He explains that the effect sunlight has on the skin depends to a large degree on the parts of the body it is allowed to strike—meaning the areas that aren't wearing clothes. Or even glasses.

"Ultraviolet light striking receptors in the retina of the eye triggers the most efficient effect on the pineal gland," he explains. "But even ordinary glass can filter out over 95 percent of the needed rays.

"To stay healthy, the main thing is to be outdoors as much as you can. Be like an animal. When it's too hot you want to stay in the shade, but when it's not, you want to have as much of your body exposed to the sun as possible. In wintertime, take advantage of warm days to let the sun hit parts of your arms that are normally covered all season. In the summer, get your sun before 10:00 A.M. and after 4:00 P.M. to avoid sunburn," says Dr. Douglass.

Among the many bodily processes that are enhanced by light on the skin, Dr. Douglass mentions that exposing your back to the sun is a most efficient way to manufacture vitamin D.

And nude sunbathers may have an energy advantage that even they never thought about. Dr. Douglass says that the genital area reacts to sunlight by manufacturing natural sex hormones within the body.

He feels that one of the reasons that the ancient Greeks were so athletically inclined is that they exercised naked. "They were naturally making the same kinds of steroids that athletes take synthetically today," he explains.

The effect of these natural steroids is to raise the levels of testosterone in the body. "And testosterone naturally makes people more energetic," says Dr. Douglass.

Fluorescent Flicker Fatigue

Take a good look at a fluorescent light. It seems to be "on" all the time, right?

Wrong. It's actually "flickering" at the rate of 60 times a second—the speed at which the charge passes between the electrodes that make the tube glow.

Although you may not be able to see the flicker, it may be perceived subconsciously and is suspected of contributing to headaches, eyestrain and our old enemy—fatigue.

Problems may diminish when regular light bulbs and/or daylight is added to the scene.

Color

Hues You Can Use

Are certain colors more appropriate for certain kinds of work? Yes, say the experts.

Red is best used for its immediate intense effect—the stimulation it supplies is great for brainstorming. To put that thinking into action, however, experts say the best color is a calm, stable one, like green.

For an institution of learning, like a college library, a combination of blue and red is recommended. The blue provides the serenity necessary for studying, while the red assures that everyone will stay awake.

Yellow, coral and orange are the recommended colors when you want to direct your energy outward, as in heavy, muscular work.

For office work, or for doing anything where you're mostly sedentary and using your mind and eyes, keep the overall brightness down and surround yourself with medium tones of green, blue-green, beige or terra-cotta. Keep most of the light source *over* what you're doing, to increase your concentration while keeping energy levels high.

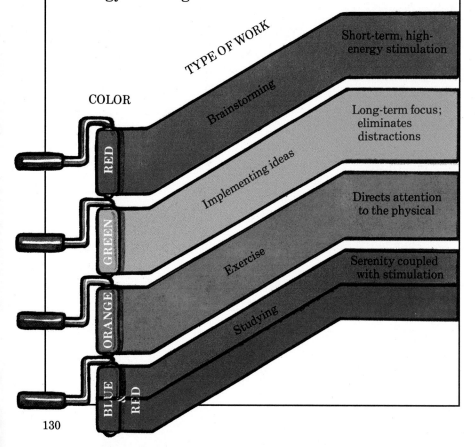

COLOR

TYPE OF WORK

ENERGY STYLE

Brainstorming — Short-term, high-energy stimulation

Implementing ideas — Long-term focus; eliminates distractions

Exercise — Directs attention to the physical

Studying — Serenity coupled with stimulation

RED · GREEN · ORANGE · BLUE · RED

Every day colors are used to manipulate you to *do* something—to buy this, use that or go there. A business specialist, writing in the trade magazine *Marketing Communications,* reminds those with something to sell that "color is a powerful persuader. The right colors can promote attention, stimulate interest, create desire and generate a favorable and positive action."

But color can also be used to your advantage. Research shows that the correct use of color can accelerate learning, retention and recall by 55 to 78 percent and increase motivation and participation by up to 80 percent.

Wouldn't you like to put colors to work for you? All it takes is a bit of understanding about the effect that color has on your energy levels.

Color's effects can be remarkably physical in nature. One of the more interesting discoveries in this field is that the color pink can act like a tranquilizer. Alexander Schauss, director of the institute for Biological Research at City College in Tacoma, Washington, has described this phenomenon in detail.

Holding a 2-foot by 3-foot piece of bright pink paper in front of people experiencing feelings of anger and frustration caused them to experience a significant loss of muscular strength. That's right, they actually became physically weaker—in a way that could be easily measured—within a period of 10 or 15 minutes.

When a similar piece of blue paper replaced the pink, the subjects' strength returned.

Unlike other environmental factors, the physical response to color is not limited to those felt to be "sensitive"—only 2 out of 153 subjects failed to experience a loss of strength when exposed to pink in one test. In another experiment, all 38 people felt a decrease in strength.

It's important to remember that the effects of bold or vibrant colors—in fact *any* color—are temporary and that the reactions subside after a short time.

In his book *Color and Human Response,* one of the most respected color authorities, Faber Birren, points out that there is an immediate—and measurable—reaction when people are exposed to a very strong hue. But like the jolt supplied by a cup of coffee, that reaction fades away—and may leave fatigue in its wake.

The color red, says Birren, is a good example. Red can raise the blood pressure and pulse rate, increase perspiration and excite brain waves. However, after a period of such intense stimulation, these bodily responses may actually respond by falling *below* normal. So for color to be used functionally, Birren says that a *variety* of colors must be used "to keep human responses continually active and to avoid visual adaption or emotional monotony."

Birren states that blue's action is the opposite of red's, lowering pulse and blood pressure, reducing the amount of perspiration and calming brain waves. Green is neutral. We react to yellow and orange much the same as to red, but not as severely. Purple and violet cause us to react much as blue does.

ALL WHITE IS NOT ALL RIGHT

Remember when your mother would come into the room and turn on all the lights, saying that reading in the dark would give you eyestrain? She may not have been doing you a favor—at least if your room had white walls.

The biggest loss of energy in the use of color occurs when brightly lit rooms and white walls combine to tire and fatigue the eyes and mind.

In the purely aesthetic sense, Birren feels that "white has little emotional appeal; it is neutral, sterile and likely to be monotonous if not boring." Health-wise, he warns that "excessive use of white on walls in such places as offices, schools and hospitals will lead to definite hazards if this white environment also includes high levels of illumination."

The "high brightness" associated with this combination causes serious visual disruption, much like the "snow blindness" encountered by skiers on a sunny day. The result is eyestrain, as voluntary muscles struggle hard against a strong reflex action to close

down the opening of the pupil. The eye tires quickly and actually loses the precision of adjustment needed to clearly see the work involved.

Birren warns that actual visual disorders and even nearsightedness can follow, "perhaps not in a day or a week, but over a prolonged period." One way to ease the problem would be to use pictures, posters or other colors to break up the mass of white surrounding you—or simply to lower the light level a bit.

Lots of color. Lots of variety. This is the color key to help us keep our energy level up and our fatigue down. But how can we manage to promote an energy "high" in environments that look the same for sometimes years on end—places like our home or workplace? Who can afford the time, money (or energy!) for routine remodeling? Luckily you don't have to. There is a middle ground.

Cooler colors should be used for work spaces, says Birren, but he urges that monotony be avoided. "Treat the eyes and human moods to moderate variety," he suggests, "and the joy of color will keep spirits high."

Birren's pick for walls is a suntan beige. Again, white or off-white is okay only for ceilings. Light colors that bring out the greatest comfort and efficiency are peach, pink, yellow, pale green and aqua, perhaps accented by coral, orange, gold, terra-cotta, green, turquoise and blue.

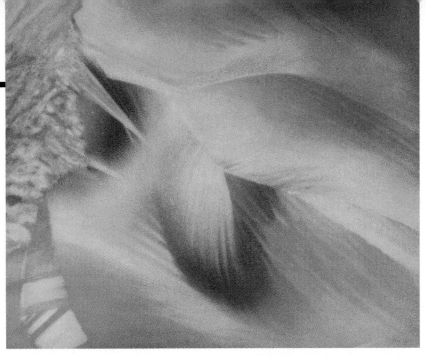

This may look like a scene from one of those psychedelic "light shows" that music groups like the Grateful Dead and the Jefferson Airplane used in the 1960s, but the members of those bands were just being born when these images were in fashion. Called Auroratone Films, the short movies were shown to mental patients suffering from psychotic depression. The shifting, swirling abstract color patterns, accompanied by slow, almost sad music, improved the moods—and the energy level—of those who watched. Attention span increased, nervous tics disappeared, and patients were calmed. One subject became "less agitated and depressed . . . more active and alert." The stimulation of the films had a positive effect on every patient who watched them.

The Workplace

When you're at home and the air seems a little stuffy, the solution is fairly simple—just open a window. But if you have the same sensation of stuffiness while working in one of those modern, energy-efficient, hermetically sealed office buildings, you'd need a brick to achieve the same result. So you sit there, powerless and frustrated.

And maybe the air *is* pretty bad. The list of indoor nasties that can show up in modern office buildings reads like a veritable "Who's Who" of fatigue felons: formaldehyde, ozone, carbon monoxide, carbon dioxide, nitrogen oxides and some 200 to 300 other contaminants that include smelly hydrocarbons as well as the ever-popular pollens, fungi and bacteria.

The number of complaints about the quality of the air in office buildings is rising rapidly—it's called the sick-building syndrome. As we seal up buildings tightly to maintain energy levels, we may wind up robbing the workers of theirs.

A large proportion of the employees of one company located in Long Island, for instance, reported after moving into their new modern building that they often felt fatigued. The symptoms got so bad that eventually more than half of the staff was working in rented trailers outside.

The problem was simply inadequate ventilation. Only half of what industry considers the normal amount of fresh air was coming into the building. Exhaust fans were installed that tripled the amount of incoming fresh air. Employees were then able to return to their former office space *and* their former energy levels.

Unfortunately, the physician who uncovered the cause warned that we can expect to see similar problems, thanks to the efforts industries are making to reduce energy consumption in such buildings.

Most of the energy-sapping side effects of today's "tight buildings" are due to inadequate fresh air and poor control over the humidity. Air conditioners and humidifiers that are regularly cleaned and disinfected, for instance, are less likely to cause respiratory problems or breed infections. So why don't the people in charge simply clean and control the air and humidity?

A Yale University study revealed that owners and employers tend to ignore complaints about their buildings. More important, it found that the people in charge really don't understand how their buildings work to begin with or what would happen to the ventilation if they made changes in office design.

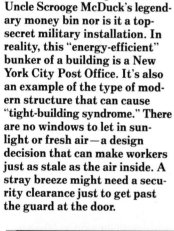

Where have all the windows gone? This is not a photo of Uncle Scrooge McDuck's legendary money bin nor is it a top-secret military installation. In reality, this "energy-efficient" bunker of a building is a New York City Post Office. It's also an example of the type of modern structure that can cause "tight-building syndrome." There are no windows to let in sunlight or fresh air—a design decision that can make workers just as stale as the air inside. A stray breeze might need a security clearance just to get past the guard at the door.

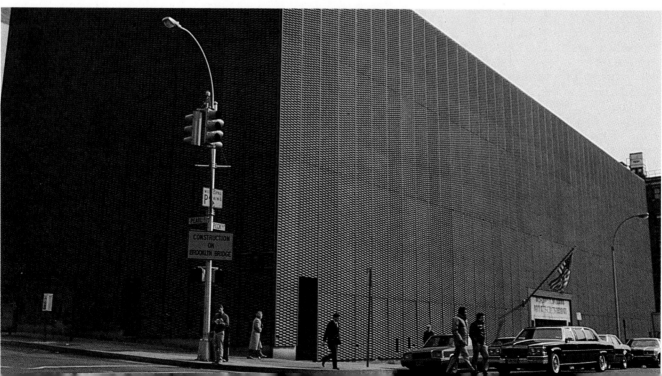

POOR ENVIRONMENT BREEDS FATIGUE

Pretty frustrating, right? Well, frustration breeds stress, and experts feel that fatigue is the direct result of the combination of the *many* stressful situations found in the modern workplace. In fact, some feel that this combination of stressors attacks our energy more directly than exposure to any individual pollutants and toxins.

Jeanne Stellman, Ph.D., and Susan Daum, M.D., make a distinction between the two types of fatigue found in the workplace. Muscle fatigue is a natural consequence of physical labor. But there's another kind of fatigue, brought on by a combination of stresses in the workplace. These include monotony, long or irregular hours, mental and physical exertion and environmental conditions such as climate, light and noise. Mental and emotional concerns—worrying about your job responsibilities or about just keeping it—add to the total. This general fatigue is characterized by feelings of boredom, weariness, depression, lassitude, anger and exhaustion. Ignore these symptoms and you may end up with a more serious condition—chronic fatigue. You'll feel tired most of the time, beaten before you start.

All of these fatiguing factors add up to *stress*—particularly if there are other problems in the office like stale air, formaldehyde leaking out of the partitions or nasty little microorganisms taking up housekeeping in the ventilator ducts.

Stress in the office is like a street gang. It wears you down by sheer weight of numbers, tiring you out until you can't defend yourself anymore. It mugs you—not for money but for your energy.

But you can fight back with "sensible work hours, rest periods, job rotations to relieve monotony and pleasant surroundings," say Dr. Stellman and Dr. Daum. "The elimination of noise is especially important in preventing fatigue in the workplace."

Friends at work are also impor-

tant. They form a necessary support group and may be able to lobby for changes that can drive some of the energy robbers out of the office environment.

Odors, for instance. A strange smell in the air signals that you may be inhaling a substance you'd rather not. The best indoor air odor is no odor at all.

Anything you do to make it seem like you have a bit more control over your personal environment at work helps to relieve the stress and restore your energy. Personal items that complement your surroundings, a window that opens, a small fan to circulate air, friendly companions, an understanding employer—all can act to fight fatigue.

How to Be Comfortable with a VDT

"Your head should not be popping out like a turtle's," explains Pat Dunphy, a physical therapist and clinical director of the HEAR (Health through Exercise and Rehabilitation) Institute in New Jersey. She's talking about the position assumed by many of the people who have computer screens (Video Display Terminals) in their school, home or workplace. "They look like someone driving through fog with their nose pressed up against the windshield," she says, adding that a more physically tiring position would be difficult to find.

This round-shouldered slouch, called the flexion position, can lead to severe muscle spasms. It causes fatigue, as well as the headaches, neck, back, shoulder and chest pain—even a sense of sinus congestion—that occur when "the lungs can't expand and you're not using any muscles," explains Ms. Dunphy.

The answer is to do what you were always told in school—sit up straight! "Sit on the edge of your chair or use a bench or one of those new 'kneeling chairs,'" says Ms. Dunphy.

But you can't fill the prescription for a perfect posture unless the video screen is at the right height. It should be at eye level when you're sitting erect with your spine nice and straight. How straight? "Watch a really good typist," says Ms. Dunphy. "She sits up *straight!*"

Ms. Dunphy also agrees with the experts who insist that VDT operators have to get away from the screen for 15 minutes every 2 hours, and she says they should spend that time walking and stretching.

Test Your Sensitivity

Are You Weather Sensitive?

To see just how much the weather outside affects your energy, take this weather-sensitivity test. Give yourself the indicated points if you answer yes to a question. Please answer *all* questions.

PHYSIQUE	POINTS
Are you lean, slender or lanky?	3
Are you of average build or muscular?	0
Are you broad, stocky or stout?	3

TEMPERAMENT	POINTS
Do you tend to be amiable, extro-verted, jolly?	1
Are you often emotionally changeable, excitable?	3
Do you tend to be acquiescent or easily led?	3
Are you often irritable or moody?	1
Do you tend to be pessimistic, easily depressed?	2
Are you often shy, inhibited, private?	3
Do you tend to be nervous?	4

SOCIOECONOMIC STATUS (APPROXIMATE)	POINTS
Are you a professional, executive, or upper class?	3
Are you middle-management or a white-collar worker?	0
Are you a blue-collar, clerical or factory laborer?	3

AGE	POINTS
Are you 10 to 19 years old?	3
Are you 20 to 29 years old?	2
Are you 30 to 39 years old?	1
Are you 40 to 49 years old?	2
Are you 50 to 59 years old?	3
Are you older?	4

SEX	POINTS
Are you female?	3
Are you male?	0

Scoring

Add up your total points and then check below to see how sensitive you are to the weather.

- A score of 0 to 5 points indicates that you are relatively *weather resistant.*
- A score of 6 to 10 points suggests you are *weather receptive* and frequently aware of your reactions to weather changes.
- If you scored 11 to 15 points, you are *weather sympathetic* and never indifferent to weather conditions.
- If you scored 16 to 20 points, you are *weather susceptible* and always in touch with the weather and its induced symptoms in you.
- With a score of 21 to 25 points, you are *weather responsive,* and every passing front is felt in your body, your moods and your behavior, which mirror the atmospheric conditions.
- A score above 25 points indicates *weather keenness,* an intense sensitivity to weather in which extreme pain or pleasure tends to accompany every weather situation. Rare individuals may experience special intense feelings in response to the weather.

Are You Environment Sensitive?

Just as with the weather, some people are more sensitive than others to the energy robbers in their surroundings. Take this simple quiz to see how big an effect the environment has on your energy levels. We've listed some environmental factors and situations. Circle the appropriate answer.

1. Do you feel less energetic when it's a smoggy day, or when pollen levels are high?
   (a) always;   (b) sometimes;   (c) never.

2. Do you have hay fever or hives?
   (a) always;   (b) sometimes;   (c) never.

3. Do you notice any irritation, allergic symptoms or actual weakness or light-headedness when you are exposed to tobacco smoke?
   (a) always;   (b) sometimes;   (c) never.

4. During the wintertime, do you always seem to be "coming down with something" —watery eyes, scratchy throat, sneezes, sniffles?
   (a) always;   (b) sometimes;   (c) never.

5. When you're indoors, do you feel more energy in the summer than in the winter? (Remember: only when you're inside!)
   (a) always;   (b) sometimes;   (c) never.

6. Are you the first to notice a new smell of any kind—either at home or at work or even when you're out with other people?
   (a) always;   (b) sometimes;   (c) never.

7. If there's a strange smell in the air (like the odor of some strong industrial cleaner or a solvent/varnish kind of smell), does it bother you?
   (a) always;   (b) sometimes;   (c) never.

8. How about a strong but pleasant smell, like perfume, air freshener, or a strongly scented soap—do these odors bother you?
   (a) always;   (b) sometimes;   (c) never.

9. Does catching a glimpse of someone wearing bright red or orange ever give you a quick surge of energy or wake you up when you're feeling a little dull?
   (a) always;   (b) sometimes;   (c) never.

10. If the winter weather keeps you indoors, do you come down with "cabin fever" or "the winter blues"?
    (a) always;   (b) sometimes;   (c) never.

11. When summer finally arrives, do you schedule yourself so that you spend as much time as possible outside in the daylight?
    (a) always;   (b) sometimes;   (c) never.

12. Do you think it's too noisy where you live?
    (a) always;   (b) sometimes;   (c) never.

13. Does the noise where you work interfere with your ability to do your job?
    (a) always;   (b) sometimes;   (c) never.

14. Do noisy appliances around the house— vacuum cleaners, washers, air conditioners, refrigerators—ever get on your nerves?
    (a) always;   (b) sometimes;   (c) never.

15. When you're tired, or even a little down, do you ever put on some music or turn on the radio to cheer up?
    (a) always;   (b) sometimes;   (c) never.

16. Are there people you deliberately avoid at work? And if they "catch you" in conversation do you feel drained afterward?
    (a) always;   (b) sometimes;   (c) never.

17. While you're at work, do you feel tired or experience headaches, sore throat, shortness of breath, burning eyes or sinus problems?
    (a) always;   (b) sometimes;   (c) never.

18. Are you physically uncomfortable at work (is it too stuffy, too bright, too noisy, too crowded, bad furniture, etc.)?
    (a) always;   (b) sometimes;   (c) never.

10

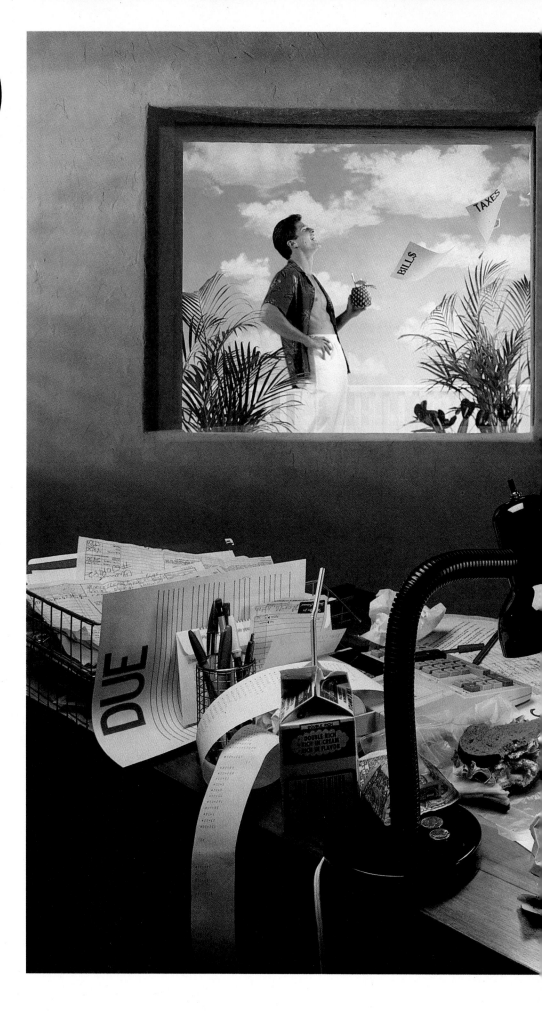

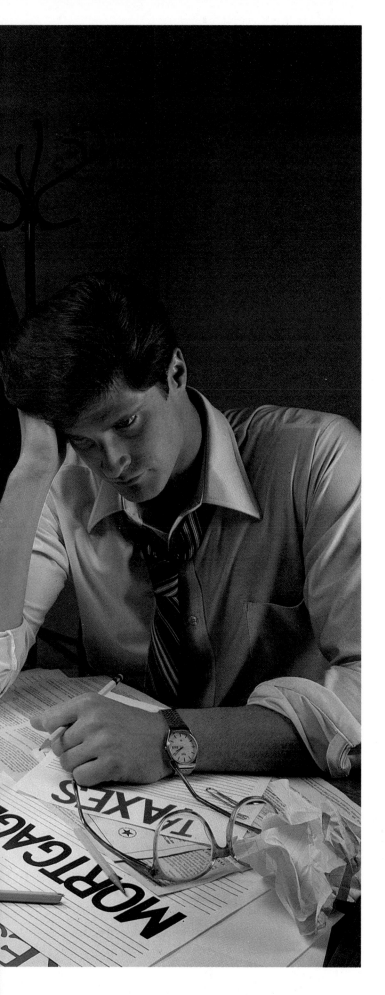

Beating Mental Fatigue

Boredom, monotony, tedium—get rid of them and you're on your way to boosting your mind power

You say your mental outlook's about as colorful as ring around the collar and as varied as a hike through a ditch? It's that old, familiar, stuck-in-a-rut syndrome. It can catch up with you in minutes as you perform a repetitious task or it can sneak up on you after years in a job that once fascinated you.

Ruts come in all shapes, sizes and walks of life. But there are ladders that each of us can use to peek over the tops of our ruts, freshen our perspectives, open our minds and spark up dull thinking.

Making that effort to peer out of your rut can pay off immediately in more variety, excitement and challenge in your daily life. It also can help open your eyes to options that had been invisible. At the least, it will enable you to perceive the world as broader and more interesting than you'd imagined.

Of course, many of us already have come up with ingenious ways to beat the everyday blahs. A jolt of exercise works miracles for many of us, whether we walk around the block or do triathlons. And we hope that you've worked out other breaks, treats and celebrations that add energy to your routine, too.

But what if some small voice nevertheless still whispers, "There must be more to life than this"? Pardon our presumption, but maybe it's time to take a look at your *thinking*.

How important is it to stay fresh mentally? One physician has written a scholarly book hypothesizing that the bored brain causes cancer. Whether or not this theory will prove true we don't know. But we do know that it's no fun to be bored. And we also know there's no need for it. You can enliven your mind—make yourself smarter and more imaginative, improve your ability to think, reason and empathize—at any age, scientists say. Thought

137

They Lead *Many* Lives

Frank Tapia is a professional photographer. Frank Tapia is an Alameda County probation officer. Frank Tapia is a runner who qualified for the Boston marathon by training 3 hours a day. And Frank Tapia is a construction worker who has done $40,000 worth of house renovations over the past 2 years. All of these statements are true. There is only one Frank Tapia. And there is nothing boring about his life.

How does he do it? "Goals," is his answer. "I always know where I want to be next, and I break it down into little steps." An example: He once called 125 ad agencies to pitch his photo work. Yield: 25 interviews and 5 people giving him regular assignments.

Concentration and the ability to switch easily from tension to relaxation is how Louise Bettner, Ph.D., claims she manages her multifaceted life. Dr. Bettner is a psychotherapist and a professional pianist who teaches both subjects. She also runs daily and is a veteran of the 7.5-mile Bay-to-Breakers race. In her spare time, she studies singing and painting and reads science fiction.

"I don't loll around much," she says. Her secret: "I love everything I do." And when problems come up, she doesn't let them fester. She clears them out of her way by dealing with them immediately so that they don't sap her energy.

processes like inductive and deductive reasoning, math skills, problem-solving ability and the capacity to spark lively new ideas can all be sharpened, no matter how old you are.

To truly open your mind, however, takes time. "It's a long process," laments Richard W. Paul, Ph.D., the director of the Center for Critical Thinking and Moral Critique at Sonoma State University in California. But it's worth the effort.

"Recognizing that you don't like it, that it's extremely uncomfortable for you to try to think in new ways, shows that it's just what you need to do," says Robert M. Bramson, Ph.D., coauthor of *The Art of Thinking.* "So give yourself a pat on the back for

trying," he says. Think of it as mental growing pains.

For instance, people who primarily think intuitively often see the act of balancing a checkbook as impossible, he says. But if you happen to be married to an analytical thinker, you *must* learn how to balance a checkbook or "your mate will never consider you a full and equal partner in decision making."

Knowing that learning how to do the checkbook will be painful and that you will not enjoy one second of it can actually be helpful, Dr. Bramson maintains. You won't be burdened by the false expectation that it should be easy for you.

Making a serious effort to expand the way you think will always involve a certain amount of discomfort, experts agree. Fair-mindedness, or the ability to see an issue from more than one side, is an ability that "people lack almost entirely," says Dr. Paul.

"People have biases and prejudices, and to have them is not to see yourself as having them. To a prejudiced person, an unprejudiced person is prejudiced," he says.

BE A SWITCH-THINKER

There is a way out of this mental morass, according to Dr. Paul. It's to consciously try to appreciate—not just acknowledge—points of view of people with whom you disagree.

Sound tough? It is. As an example of how tough it can be, he suggests trying to appreciate the communist point of view—get yourself to the point where you can understand that the other side can be right and your side may be wrong. Are you getting an idea of just how difficult changing your viewpoint can be?

But boosting your mental power doesn't mean you have to take on the world. You can begin to shake out the mental cobwebs and help yourself to a broader, fairer mind in smaller ways. For example, switch news magazines or newspapers to find out what "the other guy" has to say. Change the TV channel from soap operas to quiz shows, or from quiz shows to PBS.

And deliberately seek out speakers with whom you disagree, suggests K. Warner Schaie, Ph.D., professor of human development and psychology at Pennsylvania State University, whose research has confirmed the connection between open-mindedness and intelligence in later life. You can practice by trying to give an honest ear to politicians you don't agree with. Or by attending lectures given by controversial figures. Nearby schools may offer such events for free. You'll expose yourself to a brand new way of thinking.

In addition to throwing open your mental shutters to allow in different points of view, you can make an even more basic—and more difficult— shakeup in your thinking, says Dr. Bramson. You can change not only *what* you think but also the *way* you think. Of course, to completely alter your habitual thinking patterns would be impossible. But it *is* possible to increase your ability to use different styles of thinking.

Research shows that there are five basic thinking styles. A large percentage of us use one almost exclusively. Another large group tends to rely on one but has a backup of another one or two styles they feel comfortable with. Only a slim 13 percent of us are capable of calling on four or five patterns. You can, if you're willing to make the effort of truly expanding your mind, become one of these gifted few.

According to Dr. Bramson, if you are an *analyst,* you look for the one best way to do everything. Once you find it, you won't consider alternatives.

A *pragmatist* is always ready to try a new method, even when it's inappropriate.

Idealists like to consider everyone's wants and needs, but find it difficult to act if anyone is in opposition.

Realists view facts as being very literal. They find it virtually impossible to understand that their facts may be someone else's opinions. To realists, their own world view is it. How could anyone else see things differently?

Synthesists, on the other hand, are so adept at arguing opposing points of view that they may

have trouble settling on one of their own. As soon as they convince you, they'll swing around and defend the other side.

One desperate realist thinker and corporate executive consulted Dr. Bramson after being told that he was never going to be promoted if he didn't learn to handle people better. "That was the '2-by-4' that prompted him to undertake the difficult task of changing the way he thought," says Dr. Bramson.

After getting Dr. Bramson's advice, the executive enlisted his co-workers in a scheme to help him change. Now when he finds himself furiously pursuing a goal against resistance, his peers will remind him that other people may see things differently. He'll hear their refrain, "Shades of gray, Ken, shades of gray."

Each of the five styles of thinking has merits, insists Dr. Bramson. But you should choose your style to suit the situation. An analytically oriented wife who responds to her husband's suggestion of a romantic vacation with a list of prohibitive financial factors is using the wrong style for the occasion, Dr. Bramson says. Idealistic thinking—responding to her husband's feelings and wants— should be her first reaction.

THE NAME OF THE GAME— "THINK!"

So you want to learn new ways to think. But how? Playing games can be one simple way to improve thinking skills, say experts. Books such as *Brain Muscle Builders* by Marco Meirovitz and Paul I. Jacobs give instructions or games that can improve inductive and deductive logic, problem-solving and decision-making skills. "But," reminds Dr. Bramson, "the games that will help you the most are games you won't like. They'll fill you with tension." Idealists, for instance, will not relish games that develop analytical thinking by forcing their minds through step-by-step procedures.

Chess, a game that sharpens several styles of thinking, presents different problems to different people. Realists, for one, will have

A Long-Test Survival Guide

Grueling. That's what experts call those half-day and all-day tests like the SAT's and civil service and graduate exams. And if one of them stands between you and your goal, you want to be at your best, right to the bitter end. But how do you get your body and mind to endure it all?

Treat your body as if you were an athlete in training, advise the experts. Eat and sleep well.

Also, study old copies of the test and take sample tests until you feel comfortable with the format. It'll help get rid of those energy-draining jitters. Test-taking courses can help, particularly with specialized material like the written law boards.

Then relax and take the test, confident you'll do your best.

---

trouble with chess because "their minds move so fast they lose touch with what's happening on the board," says Dr. Bramson. But you can improve your mental skills by simply forcing yourself to go through the loathed task.

If you want to develop the analyst's ability to evaluate financial reports, for instance, first acknowledge that it does not come naturally to you. "Pat yourself on the back if you read through part of it without screaming or throwing it across the room," Dr. Bramson says. Understand that though there will be a lot of tension involved, slowly, as you persist, the task will become easier, though never pleasant, for you.

Taking a look at the way you think may also help you solve the puzzle of why you may be different from your peers, adds Dr. Bramson.

Best of all, he says, working on your thinking "frees you of the insidious perception that people who think differently from you are defective."

GETTING A NEW VIEW

Often when we have a problem, we find our minds returning to it, gnawing at it like a dog with a bone. This may be a good time to freshen your thinking by trying to see the problem from a different angle. Ask yourself if this problem has any value for you. Can you learn anything from it?

This kind of thinking can help you look at a boss who is making your life miserable with carping criticisms and say, "He is not my enemy; he is my teacher. He's teaching me how to be a good boss by showing me what a bad boss is," says psychologist Beverly A. Potter, Ph.D., author of *Beating Job Burnout*. "But at the same time he's also teaching me how to handle criticisms."

Many of us at first are reluctant to attempt this kind of mental gymnastics. We worry that seeing a situation or a person from more than one perspective is weak minded, that we're not sticking to our intellectual guns. We feel this way until we risk trying it.

"Ask yourself, 'Is this a crisis or an opportunity?' instructs Donald A. Tubesing, Ph.D., a psychologist

---

and minister who is the author of *Kicking Your Stress Habits.* Asking this question may transform a situation that was driving you crazy into a chance to grow. Dr. Tubesing refers to this process as "calling spades diamonds." It can make you see a dissatisfaction as a useful piece of information—as possibly the first step in an important change in your life.

"Most people don't know that the mind is a wild animal like an untamed elephant that must be managed," says Dr. Potter. "You can't just let it run around wherever it wants. You have to control it." And these alternative viewpoint techniques can help you harness the energies of your own mind.

One way to help tame your mental beast is to send it back to school. Take a class in something that interests you. If not much does, take a class in something that might interest you someday or that once interested you in the past. Sometimes you need to get involved before you get interested, experts say. The mental blahs may be a sign of a simple lack of activity in your life. Volunteer work might be another outlet that can give back more energy than it takes. It may give you that precious gift of seeing through another's eyes—probably someone less fortunate than yourself.

FOUR-STAR FUN

Maybe you've become caught up in doing too many things you don't like, suggests Robert Veninga, Ph.D., co-author of *The Work-Stress Connection.* You can find out if this is your problem by making a list of the things you must do today and putting a star by the ones you enjoy. Too few stars, and you can be sure life has become dull.

The answer, says Dr. Veninga, is to expand the starred activities so that they fill up more of your day. What happens, he says, is that as people get worn down, the things they don't like doing preoccupy them. Nurses who prefer caring for patients find themselves spending most of their time on hospital politics, for example.

Social psychologist Ayala Pines, Ph.D., offers an even more surefire method for breaking boredom's grip. "Write down the three things you like to do best and *do* them," she instructs.

What if you have become so calcified in your boredom that you honestly don't know what you want to do? Aim for anything at all, instructs Dr. Pines. It will help get you moving. Don't hesitate to set your sights on a star.

People are sometimes afraid to envision destinations for themselves because they're not sure it's where they really want to be. Don't worry about it, she says. Your aims are never carved in granite. They can always change.

AIM HIGH

Dr. Joyce Brothers knew just what she wanted when she was an impoverished young mother and graduate student—a Cadillac. Many people would have simply dismissed her wish as an impossible dream. But she gambled on a long shot, she recounts in her autobiography.

She reasoned that a petite blonde such as herself who became an authority on boxing would have a good chance of getting on the popular TV quiz show, "The $64,000 Question." She was right. Her appearance and victory on the program launched her career as a celebrity psychologist. And needless to say, she got her Cadillac.

Don't downgrade your dream, say experts. It'll be more motivating and energizing if you're going for the real thing, not some watered-down version of it. Where would Dr. Brothers be today if she'd decided that a used Chevy would do? If you want to be a pilot, don't settle for working at the airport.

Todd, a young man who works in his father's gas station, decided that a pilot was exactly what he wanted to be.

"It's taken longer and cost more money that I thought it would. I can't afford to get my car fixed," he says. "But wow, do I love to fly!"

Make a list of tiny steps toward your destination. Taking even one moves you a lot closer, say psycholo-

gists, because you've made a beginning. Deliberately set up positive outcomes. Buy a book on flying. It will reinforce you. Set up an appointment to take a sample lesson.

CONCENTRATION—MORE THAN A GAME

Maybe you've found that one impediment to getting where you want to be is your own wandering mind. It may just be that you're what scientists call a low screener. That's the term they've come up with for those of us who find it troublesome—or virtually impossible—to tune out the environment and concentrate on the task at hand.

When the environment contains a beautiful, sunny window, low screeners look out of it longingly. When the environment is abrasive—noisy co-workers, for instance—we grit our teeth and find it impossible to focus.

It may be small comfort, but scientists tell us that almost all artists are low screeners. Unfortunately, that is about all the comfort there is. Research indicates that your level of screening ability is inherited and is very hard to change. The solution is one that low screeners generally hate. (They actually love the distractions, it seems.) The low screener who must study or work should seek out quiet, boring, windowless environments. It's their best hope for improving concentration.

Professional athletes have perhaps the most intense interest in concentration. Perhaps even more than muscles or agility, concentration is the key to a winning game. Athletes have found that relaxation techniques—hypnosis, visualization and meditation, for instance—improve their ability to concentrate. And a calm mind is easiest to focus.

Your imagination and other mental powers are rich resources, say experts, just waiting for you to tap into them for pleasure, profit or entertainment. And just like your muscles, your imagination and other mental skills will respond to exercise. The more you use them, the stronger they grow.

How to Get a Second Mental Wind

When you feel like your intellectual get-up-and-go got up and went, don't be fooled. You still have enormous reserves of energy. That's the view of the great pioneering psychologist William James. He pointed out that in emergencies like shipwrecks people call on stores of energy they didn't know they had.

So if you find your energy failing, put in a little more effort. It may be the push that sends you over the top and coasting toward a finished project.

Job Renewal

When Joe Murphy's out on the job, almost no one is glad to see him. Murphy is a cop. When he shows up at your door, it's likely that you've just been robbed, that you're having a raucous fight with your mate or that charges have been brought against you. Despite the image of policemen as white knights, most people who meet up with cops aren't all that glad to see them.

And to tell the truth, Murphy generally isn't thrilled to see most people. "I see people at their worst," he says.

Murphy, who joined the force because he wanted to help people, found himself becoming increasingly cynical about whether people were worth helping.

But the policeman came up with an ingenious solution. He took a weekend job delivering flowers. It gave him a chance to see people with smiles on their faces who were glad to see him. Joe Murphy averted burnout. He renewed his enthusiasm for helping.

Frustrated goals and stymied ideals are one of the major reasons people burn out, experts say, whether the original goal was to nurse the sick or make better widgets.

"Cynical people—people who don't care—don't burn out," says Ayala Pines, Ph.D., a psychologist and author of *Burnout, from Tedium to Personal Growth.* And a formal job is not a requirement for burnout, she says. Wives and mothers may burn out, too.

If you find your job or situation is wearing you down, check your original expectations and hopes, suggests Dr. Pines. "You may find that they were perfectly wonderful. But how realistic are they today?" she asks.

But even a well-enjoyed job at which you feel successful can become tedious after a certain number of years. Bob, for instance, had thoroughly mastered his job as a banker. It no longer presented the challenge to him that it had when he was just out of business school. He'd begun to question the meaning of his work.

His solution was to take a year's leave to teach in an inner-city school, something he'd long been interested in doing. The year of teaching refreshed his spirit. And when he returned to the bank, recounts Beverly A. Potter, Ph.D., in *Beating Job Burnout,* he had new ideas for structuring loans to make them available to homeowners for renovation in the inner city.

Susan, a college graduate who'd taken a job as a secretary, was finding less and less energy for her job. She hated every minute of it except for the three-quarters of an hour she spent clipping business stories out of newspapers for her bosses. She asked career counselor Adele Scheele, Ph.D., author of *Skills for Success: A Guide to the Top for Men and Women,* for advice. She was told to make the most of that part of her job. Rather than turning the clips over every morning, she was to set up a system where she used the clips and other information she'd gathered for her bosses as the basis for a report she presented at the end of the week.

It wasn't long before Susan was a full-time proposal writer. A job she loved had replaced a job she'd loathed.

Arranging to spend your time on tasks you like may have equally positive effects on your position. And you'll avoid one of the most common causes of burnout—spending most of your time doing something you despise.

FOLLOW YOUR FEELINGS

What if your job blahs are less than blatant? Experts say it's not uncommon for those restless, cranky feelings to have no obvious origin. If this is the case, start a negative feelings journal, advises Dr. Potter. (Dr. Pines calls it a boredom book.) Whenever those bad feelings strike, write down the circumstances. Over time, you'll be able to focus on a pattern, whether it is a lack of positive feedback from your nitpicking boss or just too much cotton-picking work that's causing your woe.

Sometimes you may find that your very success has created problems. Your abilities have drawn more work to you than you can do. Perhaps it's time to practice that old-fashioned skill called delegation, suggests Marilyn Machlowitz, Ph.D., author of *Workaholics*. If you're not ready for full-time help, you might consider hiring temps, part-timers or project leaders.

Sometimes, concede the experts, there's just no escape, at least for a while, from a boring, tedious, deadening job whose only saving grace is its salary. And in this case, as M. F. Graham, M.D., points out in *Inner Energy*, it's the woodworking shop in your basement that you're saving for or the tuition for your night classes that keeps you motivated and energized. And getting a paycheck can be an A-number-one, valid reason for working, say authorities. Don't doubt it.

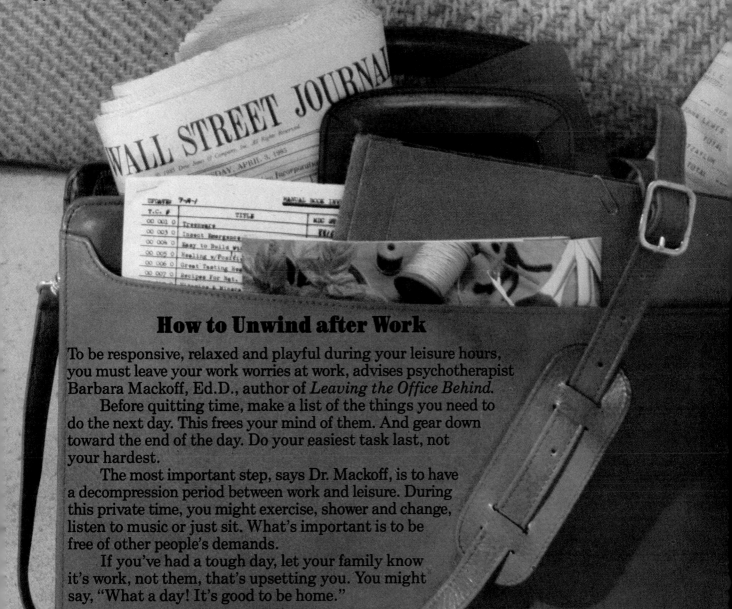

How to Unwind after Work

To be responsive, relaxed and playful during your leisure hours, you must leave your work worries at work, advises psychotherapist Barbara Mackoff, Ed.D., author of *Leaving the Office Behind*.

Before quitting time, make a list of the things you need to do the next day. This frees your mind of them. And gear down toward the end of the day. Do your easiest task last, not your hardest.

The most important step, says Dr. Mackoff, is to have a decompression period between work and leisure. During this private time, you might exercise, shower and change, listen to music or just sit. What's important is to be free of other people's demands.

If you've had a tough day, let your family know it's work, not them, that's upsetting you. You might say, "What a day! It's good to be home."

11

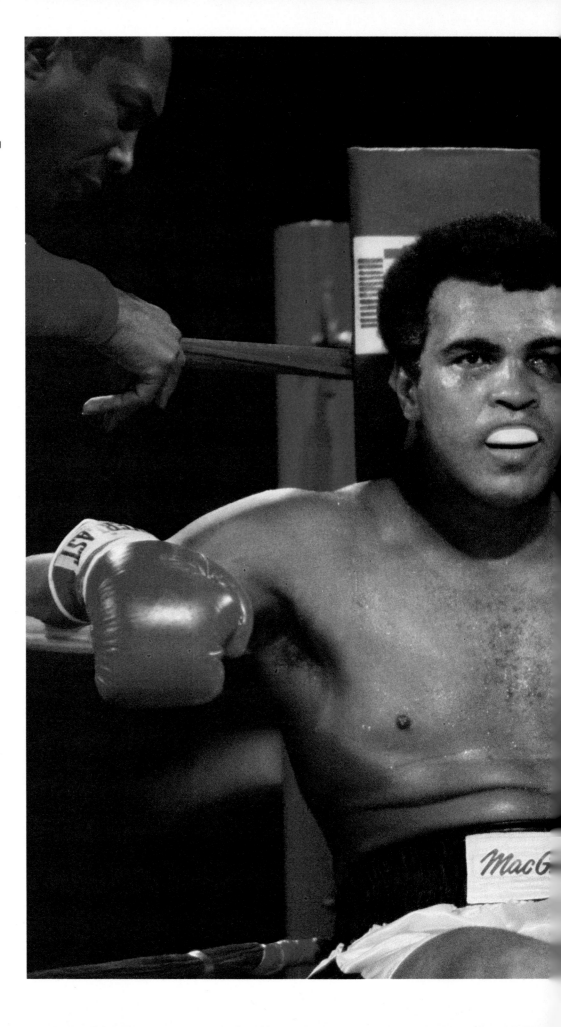

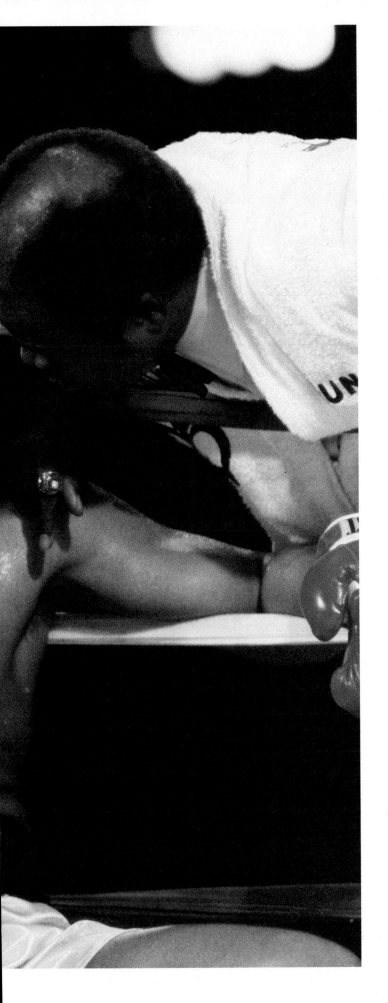

Battling Body Fatigue

Silent illnesses deep within the body can drain your energy. Here's how to knock them out!

On a torrid October evening in 1980, Muhammad Ali ducked into the ring for the final major battle of his illustrious career. But something was wrong. Ali neither floated like a butterfly nor stung like a bee. His body seemed completely drained of energy.

It wasn't age that stopped the 38-year-old champion that evening, it was a drug—Thyrolar. The champ was unaware of the crippling side effects, which led to his fatigue, weakness and intolerance to heat. He had been taking a double dose of the medication, commonly prescribed to boost a sluggish thyroid. It was 100°F in the ring that evening. Ali never had a chance.

A tragic error, but what does it mean to you? You're not planning to duke it out with any 220-pound professional fighters.

Chances are, however, that you routinely enter much deadlier arenas, where 3,000-pound chunks of steel whiz by at speeds of 60 miles per hour. Or maybe all that face you are meetings, the kind in which snap judgments can make or break you and your firm.

Wait a minute. You're not on Thyrolar. What's the point?

Did you take a sleeping pill last night? Did you wake up with the sniffles and pop the usual cold tablet? Are you on allergy capsules? Blood pressure medication? What about any of the hundreds of drugs that can leave you deadened, numbed and listless?

Don't take pills? Colds, flu or similar "walking" illnesses can also drag you down.

In today's world, the opponents waiting to tap your energy grow more formidable. This chapter will teach you to tie on the gloves and fight body fatigue.

Allergies

You know all about allergies, right? Come close to something the old body doesn't like and you start sneezing, the eyes water, the nose runs. Move away from the offending substance (or toss the offending critter outdoors) and the symptoms stop. Allergy in a nutshell.

Hold on. What about the drained feeling you get in the winter? The severe case of afternoon blahs at work? Your depression? Lack of ambition? Moodiness? These are all symptoms of allergy-induced fatigue—the Sneezeless Allergy. "Fatigue is one possible symptom of food allergy reaction," states James C. Breneman, M.D., a food allergy pioneer and author of *Basics of Food Allergy.* "Allergy is the most common cause

The Four Seasons of Fatigue

Allergies, like visits from relatives, tend to be seasonal. You may have great autumns and lousy, drowsy summers because of season-specific allergies. Spring may be your time for romance simply because the substance that fagged you out all winter has left town. Below are seasonal fatigue-inducing allergens to watch out for.

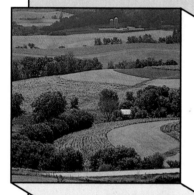

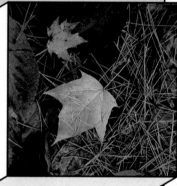

Chlorinated
  pools
Grass/weed pollen
Clogged A/C ducts
Suntan lotion
Rainy-season molds
Insect bites
Smog

Hay/grain fields
Burning leaves
Starting home heaters
Compost/leaf piles
Mothballs
Woodpiles

Summer

Fall

Spring

Winter

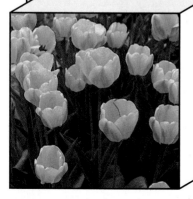

Tree/flower pollens
Flower fragrances
Spring cleaning/dusts
Cleaning fluids
Floor wax/furniture
  polish
Scouring powders
House dust mites

Fuel oil heaters
Fireplaces
Christmas trees
Hand/face creams
Weather-sealed houses
Dry gas heat

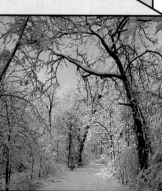

of otherwise unexplained fatigue in children." adds William G. Crook, M.D., of Jackson, Tennessee. And food isn't the only problem. Pollens and other allergens may cause fatigue, too. But *how* does allergy cause fatigue? While the skin, nose and lungs remain the most commonly recognized areas for allergies to attack, the more sneaky, insidious varieties dig deeper. The muscles, brain, joints and blood are all vulnerable to energy-sapping allergies. Therein lies a problem. Without the runny nose, the Sneezeless Allergies are frequently overlooked by doctors who, in trying to cure your fatigue, spend time, effort and wads of your money chasing the figurative wild goose instead of a literal one that left its highly allergenic feathers in your pillows.

Yet, as we pointed out, it's usually not where you bed but what you're fed that causes allergic fatigue. Unfortunately, nearly everything you eat can be suspect. Thankfully, scientists have narrowed the list down a more manageable top 21.

"Cow's milk is the worst for creating all the allergic symptoms, especially those involving fatigue and emotions," Dr. Breneman says.

Aside from milk, the remaining 20 potential pepbusters are wheat, corn, coffee, cane sugar, eggs, beef, potatoes, pork, oranges, carrots, tomatoes, yeast, apples, chicken, lettuce, soy products, peanuts, green beans, oats and chocolate.

Now that we know the suspected enemy, the next step is learning how to beat it. For food allergies, doctors differ in their methods but agree on the task—identify and banish. The ways to achieve this include fasting for a few days; limiting yourself to the least allergenic foods, mainly green and yellow vegetables, fish and fowl; or embarking upon a rare-food diet by eating foods you don't normally eat. In all three methods, the second step is to slowly reintroduce your normal diet, watch for symptoms and keep an eye out for suspected or frequently eaten foods. Whatever method you try, Dr. Breneman says the key is to be aware of the other symptoms besides fatigue. These

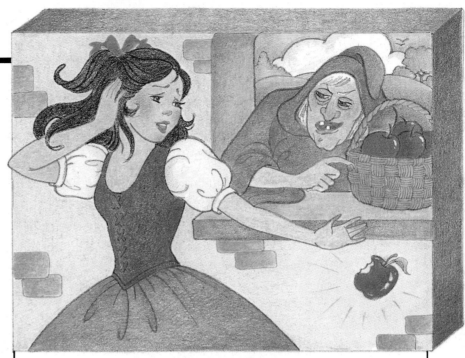

Was Snow White's Apple Really Poisoned?

Probably. But had the Wicked Witch done her homework, she might have saved on the poison potion supply. If the stunning Ms. White was allergic to apples, the apple itself might have induced a good snooze (or at least a bout of intense tiredness): One common symptom of food allergy is fatigue. And the odds were in the Wicked Witch's favor. Marshall Mandell, M.D., in his book *5-Day Allergy Relief System,* puts apples in his top 21 food allergy hit list.

What about Snow White's diminutive buddies, the Seven "Allergic" Dwarfs? We presented their sad case to the nation's most renowned food allergist, James C. Breneman, M.D.

"Sleepy, Sneezy, Grumpy, Dopey and Bashful all had symptoms of food allergies," Dr. Breneman chuckled. "If Doc could have identified and removed the troublesome foods, all the dwarfs could have been named Happy."

include hives, asthma, heartburn, abdominal cramps, gas, headaches, confusion, forgetfulness, depression, canker sores in the mouth, and aching muscles, joints or back.

For nonfood allergies, the goal is the same. Watch for symptoms, identify the culprit, then banish it from your life. If it's too common to duck, consult your doctor for medicinal help.

Anemia

nemia. Fatigue, Even Webster has given up trying to separate the words: The dictionary lists "lack of vitality" as the second official definition of anemia.

The reason, of course, is that anemia and fatigue are intertwined. If you are anemic, you're tired and run-down, a simple cause-and-effect relationship. In fact, simplicity is a key. Anemia is simple to get, usually simple to diagnose and cure. So why do millions of people have it? Simple. It's also simple to overlook. As you've been learning in chapter 10 and in this chapter, fatigue has a multitude of causes. It's no wonder so many anemics go untreated.

In short, anemia is usually caused by a lack of iron in the blood. Iron is needed to make hemoglobin, which jets oxygen to our tissues and cells, energizing them. If the iron level drops, so do hemoglobin and energy. Some cases, though, aren't quite so routine. Doctors have identified a host of other causes, including deficiencies of the B complex vitamins B_{12}, folate and riboflavin (vitamin B_2) and of vitamin C. Even "deficient" running shoes have been blamed!

As you can see by the chart below, anemia has earned its reputation as the "woman's disease." The culprit is menstruation. Blood loss means iron loss. Combine this with

Anemia: Who Has It; How to Beat It

Feeling spent? If you spot yourself in the high-risk chart, help may be as close as your supermarket.

Proper diet is the cure for most anemics. This chart shows those most likely to be anemic and lists some foods suited to their lifestyles or particular needs. Research has shown that eating foods rich in vitamin C along with high-iron foods helps the body absorb iron better. Thus, the first 3 foods in each list are high in iron, while the last supplies vitamin C.

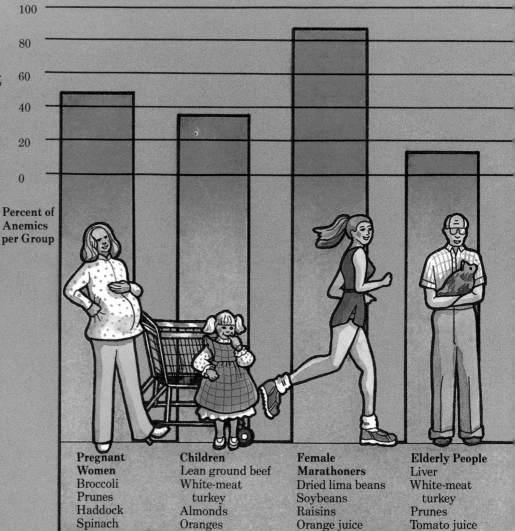

Percent of Anemics per Group

Pregnant Women	Children	Female Marathoners	Elderly People
Broccoli	Lean ground beef	Dried lima beans	Liver
Prunes	White-meat turkey	Soybeans	White-meat turkey
Haddock	Almonds	Raisins	Prunes
Spinach	Oranges	Orange juice	Tomato juice

other female stress factors such as pregnancy and birth control pills and the risk goes through the roof.

If that's not enough, toss in the burden of today's ideal of beauty.

"Any woman who owns a TV or opens a magazine is slapped with the not-so-subtle pressure to be thin, thin, thin," says Estelle Miller, founder of the American Anorexia and Bulimia Association, an organization that steps in when dietary anemia reaches the deadly self-starvation anorexic state.

"I've been shouting about those role models since 1978," adds psychotherapist Steven Levenkron of New York. "They have taught women to hate the normal female body!"

The cures for the anemia blahs are again rather simple. If your pep is pooped, have your doctor order a full-scale blood chemistry test, paying particular attention to levels of hemoglobin. Then, if the missing ingredient is iron, drag yourself to the supermarket and stock up on the right foods. For openers, beef liver, blackstrap molasses, beef, lima beans, sunflower seeds, dark-meat turkey, dried apricots, raw broccoli, spinach, almonds, peas and white-meat chicken will boost your iron. (If your doctor prescribes an iron supplement, though, *take it,* even though you may have to put up with a little constipation.)

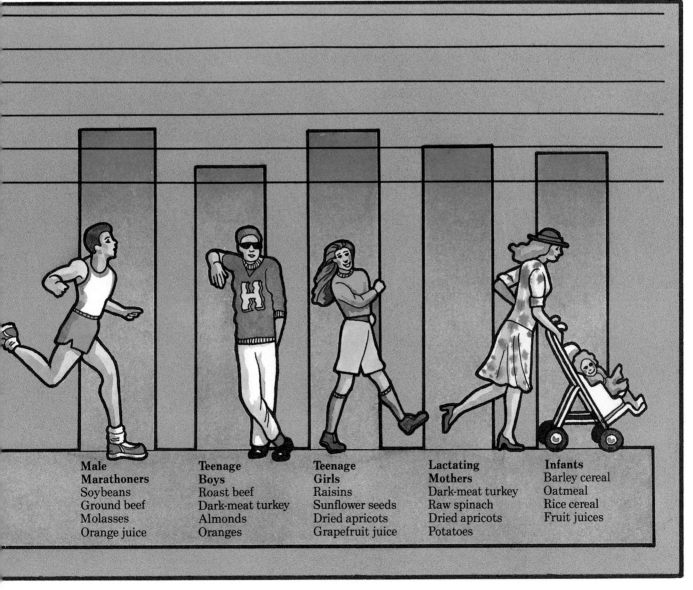

Male Marathoners	Teenage Boys	Teenage Girls	Lactating Mothers	Infants
Soybeans	Roast beef	Raisins	Dark-meat turkey	Barley cereal
Ground beef	Dark-meat turkey	Sunflower seeds	Raw spinach	Oatmeal
Molasses	Almonds	Dried apricots	Dried apricots	Rice cereal
Orange juice	Oranges	Grapefruit juice	Potatoes	Fruit juices

Circulatory Problems

In the previous pages you learned that the chemical content of blood can invigorate or drag down the body. Iron is needed to build the convoy that freights oxygen to our tissues and cells. Without the iron, fatiguing anemia results.

But what if your blood is all juiced up with nowhere to go? What if the convoy trucking energizing, revitalizing oxygen is snarled in traffic? That's what happens in your arteries and veins when you get too *much* of fatty, high-cholesterol foods like marbled steaks, ice cream and greasy french fries, and too *little* fat-burning exercise. A gooey mess of circulatory grease rides bumper to bumper inside your veins and arteries. The blood flow is reduced to a crawl. So, in turn, are you.

If a poor diet and a lazy lifestyle caused the traffic jam, chances are the fatigue will linger. And surgery isn't always the answer.

"Surgery can help only blood vessels in the area operated on," explains Robert Lowenberg, M.D., a retired vascular surgeon. "If I perform a bypass in someone's left leg—at great cost—I haven't done anything for the right leg, or the aorta, or the renal artery, or the brain."

Which explains why so many sufferers of atherosclerosis (hardening of the arteries) get little relief and remain fatigued, despite a painful operation. It also explains why so many sufferers repeat the surgery.

Left untreated, the clogged traffic can eventually close down the road altogether. That's when the heart attack hits, often resulting in the ultimate fatigue—death. Fortunately, the physical fatigue and occasional pain of a closing artery usually gives fair warning. Unfortunately, too many ignore it.

Atherosclerosis isn't the only cause of circulatory fatigue. It can be attributed simply to physical inactivity. A body stuck in first gear causes reduced blood flow, which can "starve" your body and brain of energizing fuels. An irregular heartbeat can also interfere with blood flow.

Another major problem is clots. Blood clots, like the "gremlins" in the hit movie, are good guys gone bad. Clots are caused in part by platelets—the good guys that seal up cuts and wounds and keep you from bleeding to death from minor scratches. No one's sure why they sour, but doctors know too well what happens when they do. They begin to gang up, sticking together in a glob that grows lazy and decides to hang out permanently on an artery wall. You need a medical dictionary to take it from there. Thrombosis results from a clot which can form anywhere in the arteries or veins. Phlebitis is an inflammation of the vein. A pulmonary embolism results from a clot in the lungs. A stroke can be caused by a clot in the brain. If you have clots and fatty buildups in the coronary artery, it could be heart attack time.

Wherever this "bad blood" settles, fatigue can be an early warning. Heed it!

As you can gather, there's a lot of trouble lurking in "Red River" City, trouble with a capital T that stands for Tired.

Now turn on the lights and dash the despair. Even in the worst cases of atherosclerosis, there are things

The stronger your heart and circulation, the faster the heart beats, right? Dead wrong. The heartbeat irony is that the healthier you are, the *lower* the resting heart rate. Research shows that persons with slower heart rates are 2 to 3 times less likely to die of coronary heart disease than are people with faster resting rates. The chart shows the differences between resting heart rates of peak-condition marathon runners, a nonathlete in good shape, and someone courting cardiac disaster.

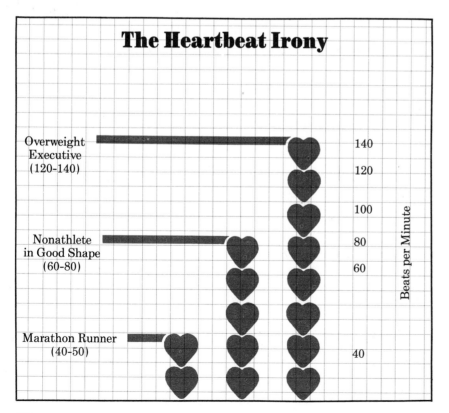

The Heartbeat Irony

Overweight Executive (120-140)

Nonathlete in Good Shape (60-80)

Marathon Runner (40-50)

Beats per Minute

140
120
100
80
60
40

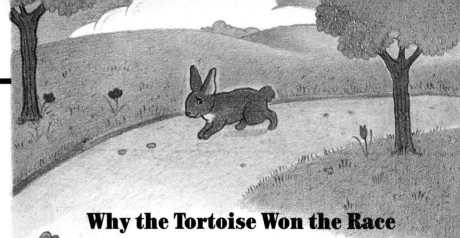

you can do to unsnarl the jam.

To start off, let's recall what the circulatory system is. It brings oxygen and fuel to the tissues and organs of the body and washes away waste. Think of it as a high-pressure water hose scouring the body from the inside. The stronger it flows, the more refreshed and cleaned out you feel. The way to rev the blood is to rev the body. Jog, walk, roller skate, join the company basketball team or a local fitness club, do aerobics, do something! You'll feel better and have more energy and, better yet, some of those early clots and fat globs may get swept away before they bunch up.

Doctors recommend 20 to 30 minutes of heart-pumping exercise three or four times a week. Jog if you can. But walking is a fine substitute if you find other forms of aerobics are not to your liking.

"Exercise builds up collateral blood vessels. These are little blood vessels the size of a hair or two that enlarge and take over the function of blocked vessels," according to one doctor. Results can begin to show up after only three weeks. "You become more alert, more interested, because now you are able to be more active. Patients feel that now there's a point to going on and living," he says.

However, exercise alone won't do the job of keeping arteries healthy. Diet is just as important. But diet is a double-edged steak knife. There are good and bad things to eat. What you'll want to do is double up on the good and cut back on the bad. Here's the formula doctors are now recommending for a healthy heart.

Drink alcohol in moderation and cut back on your intake of saturated fats and overly processed foods. Replace them with plenty of fresh vegetables, lean meats, whole grains and fruit. Give up cigarettes—forever.

A third step in fighting circulatory fatigue is to pad your diet with foods that contain the vitamins and minerals research has shown to be healthy for the heart. Magnesium, for one, helps open blood vessels in the heart tissues. Too little chromium has been linked to hardened arteries. And the old standby, vita-

Why the Tortoise Won the Race

he classic story. The silly rabbit dozed off and let the pokey tortoise win. What Aesop never explained was *why*. Medical science has a clue. Rabbits are extremely susceptible to atherosclerosis. The hardened arteries induce fatigue. Thus, the infamous "sleeping bunny" may not have been so cocky—or healthy—after all!

Today, fatigued rabbits hold greater significance. Because of their easily induced circulatory problems, rabbits have aided research for nearly a century. Many of the current methods of battling circulatory illnesses can be directly attributed to rabbits. So the next time you hear about the victorious tortoise and the vanquished rabbit, don't laugh. Tip your hat to the creature that may one day contribute to a much greater victory—beating atherosclerosis.

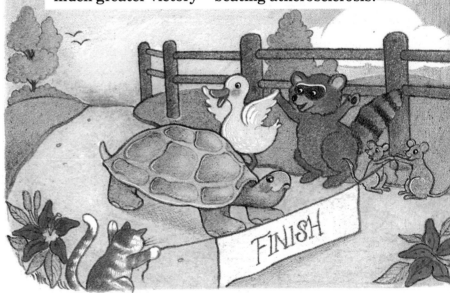

min C, has been shown to battle the evil trio of cholesterol, atherosclerosis and heart disease.

In summary, grab a vitamin/food chart, jog down to your local supermarket and load up on vitamin-rich, low-fat foods that help scrub your circulatory system and keep you going and flowing.

Diabetes

Don't turn that page! We know what you're thinking. "This is a section I can skip. Diabetes is a *major* disease. If I have it, I know it. If I don't know it, I don't have it."

It's a common, often tragic, misconception that diabetes, like the flu, is a wham-bam disease that announces itself billboard-style. The Diabetes Research Institute at the University of Miami Medical School estimates that five million Americans have it and don't know it. The reason? Fatigue, a major symptom, is a symptom of scores of other ailments and is frequently overlooked.

There are actually two types of diabetes and with both, fatigue is a major symptom. That's because diabetes interferes with the body's ability

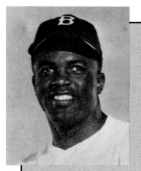
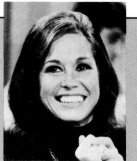
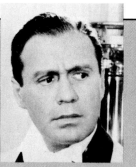
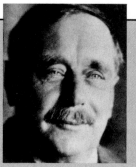
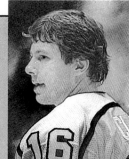

There's No Time for Fatigue

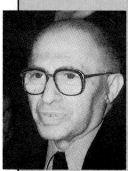
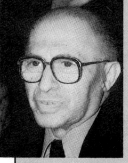
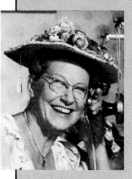
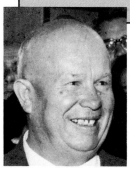

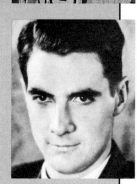
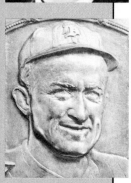

Diabetes didn't keep Elvis Presley from becoming "The King"; Jackie Robinson out of baseball's Hall of Fame; Spencer Tracy from making more than 70 movies; Mary Tyler Moore out of two hit TV series; Jack Benny from being stingy or funny; Menachem Begin from governing Israel; Bobby Clark from excelling at professional hockey; Bobby Jones out of professional basketball; Ty Cobb from getting 4,000 hits in pro baseball; Thomas Edison from lighting up the world; Ernest Hemingway from writing *The Old Man and the Sea;* Howard Hughes from making money; Nikita Khrushchev's iron hand from running Russia; Minnie Pearl from getting laughs at the Grand Old Opry; or H.G. Wells from taking us into a fantastic future.

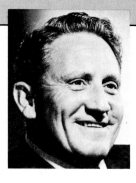
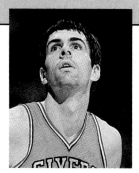
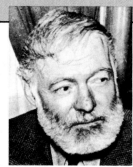
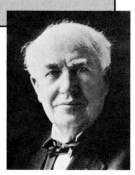

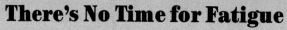

to burn sugar for energy. Type I, formerly called juvenile-onset diabetes, is the most severe form—the "I know I've got it" diabetes. The pancreas is the villain here, failing to produce the amount of insulin needed to burn sugar for energy. No insulin, no energy. Daily insulin shots are needed. Although it's the most publicized, Type I afflicts a mere 10 percent of America's 13 million diabetics.

Type II is the sneaky diabetes, the one that's easily misdiagnosed. It hits later in life, around age 40, and can be caused by being over-weight, eating poorly and sitting on your duff for a decade or two. The jury is still out on whether the pancreas is guilty here. It's producing, but the insulin no longer works. The result is the same as if you didn't have insulin—no sugar burned equals no energy.

Both Type I and Type II can do more than deplete your energy. Together, they cause the deaths of 300,000 Americans a year. Fatigue is usually one of the first warning signs. If you're whipped and suspect diabetes, be aware of the other symptoms. Frequent urination, thirst, nausea and uncontrollable craving for sweets are symptoms of Type I. Blurred vision, numbness or cramps in the legs, feet and fingers and skin infections are progressive symptoms of Type II. Blindness, high blood pressure, gangrene and loss of limbs are late-stage nightmares. Diabetes can even lead to heart attack, stroke and kidney failure.

Pretty relentless, isn't it? But it doesn't have to be that way. Thanks to advances in natural healing, Type II sufferers can restore their energy and almost obliterate their problem. The key is proper diet and exercise.

For quick reference, remember the four F's of fighting diabetic fatigue—fiber, fruit, fructose and fat. Get lots of the first three and get rid of the fourth and you're well on your way to feeling good.

Back up a letter and get E for exercise. One study has shown neglected muscle cells lose their ability to energize with insulin. Exercise in itself is a natural energizer, so the effect of the insulin is doubled!

High Fiber Equals High Energy

One key to dumping diabetic drowsiness is high-fiber foods. These "bulky" energy boosters ease sugar into the bloodstream at a rate diabetics can handle. Some doctors recommended 45 to 60 grams per day for diabetics. (Remember, however, that fiber is so effective it can lower insulin requirements— check with your doctor before embracing this diet regimen.) Below are some of the best high-fiber foods.

Food	Portion	Total Dietary Fiber (g.)
Kidney beans, cooked	½ cup	9.6
Pinto beans, cooked	½ cup	9.6
White beans, cooked	½ cup	7.9
Prunes, dried	5 medium	6.8
Spinach, cooked	½ cup	5.7
Almonds	¼ cup	5.1
Raisins	½ cup	4.9
Blackberries	½ cup	4.5
Pear	1 medium	4.0
Peas, cooked	½ cup	4.0
Corn, cooked	½ cup	3.9
Lentils, cooked	½ cup	3.7
Peanuts	¼ cup	3.4
Apple	1 medium	3.3
Sweet potato, raw	1 medium	3.3
Banana	1 medium	3.1
Potato, raw	1 medium	3.1
Broccoli, cooked	½ cup	3.0
Whole wheat bread	2 slices	2.6
Beets, sliced, cooked	½ cup	2.1
Squash, summer, cooked	½ cup	2.0
Zucchini, sliced, raw	½ cup	2.0
Brussels sprouts, raw	½ cup	1.9
String beans, raw	½ cup	1.9
Broccoli, raw	½ cup	1.6
Strawberries	½ cup	1.6
Carrots, grated, raw	½ cup	1.5
Plums	1 medium	1.4

A duo of minerals, chromium and magnesium, is your next weapon. Chromium appears to increase the effectiveness of the body's insulin in regulating blood sugar levels. Magnesium combats one of the most frightening complications of diabetes, blindness.

On the vitamin front, thiamine and vitamins C and E can help beat fatigue and fight other effects of diabetes. Thiamine helps ease the foot ailments (burning, itching, numbness) that frequently accompany the disease.

Finally, if you smoke—quit. Nicotine increases circulatory problems, and circulatory problems in diabetics are what can kill.

Drug Side Effects

Each year billions of dollars are spent on drugs that effectively mask minor discomforts while just as effectively slowing down our bodies and reflexes. There are more than a hundred antihistamines alone on the market, and almost all of them induce fatigue. On top of that, Americans spend $43 million a year on over-the-counter sleeping pills. Toss in the other OTC and prescription drugs that warn of drowsiness—blood pressure pills, painkillers, premenstrual discomfort tablets, sedatives, motion sickness pills and—ZZZZzzzzzzz— we've become a nation of nappers.

In the opening of this chapter you read the tragic story of how Muhammad Ali suffered a terrible beating in one of his last fights because a thyroid drug stripped his energy and left him virtually defenseless. Incredibly, a similar mistake nearly clouded the 1985 Super Bowl. Miami Dolphin quarterback Dan Marino had an unprecedented year, breaking nearly every passing record there was. Nothing could stop him. Nothing but a tiny red capsule. A few days before the big game, Marino suffered a brief dizzy spell before practice that sent him retreating to the bench. At first he thought it was jet lag. Team doctors finally traced the problem to a drug called Feldene, a common anti-inflammatory the great quarterback had been taking for an injured knee. Feldene, which Marino took on an empty stomach, has a host of side effects, including wooziness and gastric upset. And regardless of when you take it, "somnolence" is a listed side effect. Marino's problem was caught in time but the point is dramatically illustrated—if million-dollar athletes surrounded by the best doctors can make such mistakes, what chance do you have? You may be facing your own Super Bowl one day, be it a job interview, an entrance exam or a sales presentation, and accidentally enter the "arena" woozy and defenseless.

Why is this happening? Part of the problem is that some doctors may neglect to explain a drug's side effects, especially when they're as "routine" as fatigue. The solution here is simple: *Ask the doctor.* And after he answers, get the world's cheapest second opinion—read the federally mandated material that comes with the medication. If it's a prescription drug, ask your pharmacist for the material. If it's an over-the-counter drug, read the section on the box or in the enclosure clearly marked "Warning." The key word to ferret out is "drowsiness." If the phrase is "if drowsiness occurs," count on it! If you still need the relief, be aware of the other symptoms—depression, forgetfulness and even loss of sex drive. A good precaution is to take the drugs at night prior to sleep, or when you're taking a day off and can nap on the couch.

"But what choice do I have?" you wail. "I have horrible hay fever. Atomic headaches. My blood pressure's up, my sleep's down, I'm too hyper and my arthritis is killing me. *I need my pills!!!!!!*"

If this is you, there are some ways to avoid compounding the fatigue. But before we get into that, Joe Graedon, author of *The People's Pharmacy,* sets the record straight.

"What you must remember is there is no way to counter the drowsiness of these medications once you've taken them," he says. "You have to ask yourself, 'Do I have to live with the drowsiness?' The answer is yes. You have to pay the price. You weigh the benefits against the risk, and you and your doctor must decide if you should take the medication. It's a tough decision."

The attack plan, then, is to avoid additional fatiguing factors that may intertwine with the drugs. This includes getting a good night's sleep and eating a proper diet.

"Anything else that would make you more drowsy should be avoided." Graedon advises. "If eating a big lunch generally makes you sleepy, you might want to have a lighter lunch when you are taking these medications."

You should also be aware of the

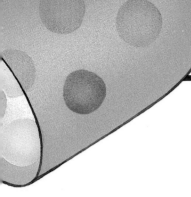

different types and strengths of the drugs. The duration of the drowsiness can vary widely with the drug, anywhere from 2 to 20 or more hours, depending on such things as your diet and how long you have taken the drug. In general, time-release pills have a longer-acting effect; if you take these medications in the morning, you may be somewhat mentally numb for anything from several hours to several days, depending on your individual tolerance.

There are also different chemicals in similar medications to be aware of. Hay fever medications come in three antihistamine types— the alkylamines, the ethanolamines and the ethylenediamines. The alkylamines have the least sedative effect, while the ethanolamines have the most. The ethylenediamines fall in between.

"The susceptibility to drowsi-ness seems to be inherent in the individual," says Graedon. "I would suggest trying different types to find the one that's the least sedating for you."

A major consideration is to "know thy enemy." Don't confuse a cold with hay fever. Antihistamines have no effect on a cold.

An obvious warning is don't double up with sedation-inducing drugs such as alcohol, tranquilizers and barbiturates.

Allergy sufferers can sidestep drowsiness altogether by using Seldane (terfenidine), the first in a new generation of nonsedating antihistamines. Consult your doctor or pharmacist.

If you need an occasional sleeping pill, a new, shorter-acting tablet called Halcion has hit the market. This may help beat the common sleeping pill hangover that can linger for up to 10 hours after you wake up.

"The important thing to remember is that the side effects of the drugs are not necessarily dangerous," says Jeremy H. Thompson, M.D., of UCLA. "It's not knowing what the side effects are that can be dangerous."

The Ten Most Common Knock-Out Drugs

Over-the-Counter
Pain relievers
Cough/cold remedies
Allergy/hay fever/
    asthma preparations
Sleeping pills
Motion sickness pills

Prescription
Heart disease drugs
Tranquilizers
Antiarthritics
High blood pressure pills
Antihistamines

Beware of Drugs That Drowse

Drugs that cause drowsiness can:
• impair driving ability.
• induce confusion and unsteadiness.
• dull thinking and memory.
• bring on depression.
• promote restlessness, irritability and headache.
• deflate sex drive or performance.
The effects can linger for 20 hours and are increased with the use of alcohol.

Flu, Colds, Infections

Ah, sweet memories of high school. The football team. Cheerleaders. Your first old bomb car. Friends you would die for. Your first girlfriend or boyfriend. Your first kiss. Your first kiss in the back seat of your old bomb car. Kissing. Kissing? The Kissing Disease! Mono. Argghhhh!

Remember mononucleosis? If you're one of the millions of Americans who've had it, you remember, all right. If you had it during high school or college, your memories of that golden period are clouded by the two months of sheer, bedridden, missing-all-the-fun agony. It was *adios* to kissing. You could have looked like Paul Newman or Victoria Principal and no one would get near you for at least six months! And the *fatigue*. We're talking killer fatigue here, endless fatigue, a fatigue that can linger for nearly a year.

This journey back to school days vividly demonstrates the fatiguing aspect of viral infections. Even if you escaped mono back in your raccoon-coat or poodle-skirt days, virtually no one escapes its less devastating but much more common viral cousins—the common cold and the flu. Both zero in on the body's energy supply, plundering it unmercifully. Even when they leave, they leave you drawn and beat, as if you'd been through a major battle—which, on a microscopic scale, you have. As far back as 1870, the great Louis Pasteur discovered that the weaker and more run-down you are, the greater your chance of contracting more infectious diseases—and getting more fatigued. Round and round it goes.

THE BAD BUG BLUES

Since a flu whips you right out, the tiring aspects are generally dealt with immediately—you collapse into bed. Some low-level "walking" flus and pneumonias do exist, but the energy drain is such that you, and everyone else, can easily identify the affliction. Also, flus, like rats, travel in packs. Chances are a half dozen co-workers or buddies have it, or just shook it (probably onto you!). This leaves the little guy, the devious cold, to do the most damage when it comes to straight fatigue. The reason is that many people just grit their teeth and bear it, taking little if any time from their daily functions to wait it out. The danger here, as with all fatigue, is that you're performing your normal functions with subnormal ability. (And so are most of your friends, since the gleefully reproductive little germs were probably spread all over.)

This is just what happens after the cold rears its homely head. A cold virus can take up to a week to incubate, and feeling out of sorts is one of the first warnings of tissues to come. Thus, a two-day cold may actually have bled the body's energy for two weeks!

So, at the first sign of a cold, you run to the drugstore and buy the killer cold tablet you saw on TV, right? Caught you! You didn't read

---

Herpes Family Branching Out

Imagine an illness that combines the resistance of herpes with the severe fatigue and ravaging symptoms of mononucleosis. Researchers at the National Institute of Allergy and Infectious Diseases (NIAID), in Bethesda, Maryland, recently associated the despised Epstein-Barr virus, the herpes virus family member that causes mononucleosis, with a devastating illness that can debilitate its victims for as long as 5 years. The newly recognized disease, currently called chronic mononucleosis, has yet to be formally named.

"People with this illness are not as sick as with mononucleosis, but it can last much longer," says NIAID researcher Stephen Straus, M.D. "The real problem is its main symptom, chronic fatigue, is so common the disease is often overlooked."

Dr. Straus adds that 90 percent of Americans are exposed to Epstein-Barr by age 30, but only a very small (presently undetermined) percentage are chronically afflicted.

Those who suspect they have this disease should ask their doctor to test for mononucleosis. Doctors should be aware that this strain is harder to detect because its symptoms aren't as severe.

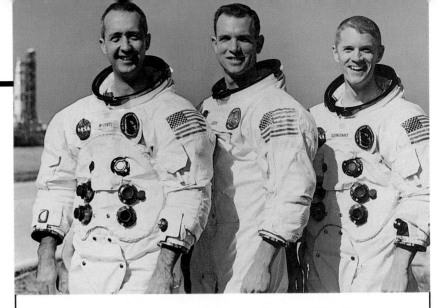

the previous information on drugs. If you had, you would have learned that some types of over-the-counter cold medications contain antihistamines that make you drowsy—the last thing you need when you're already half zonked. Antihistamines can also clog up the mucus in your air passages and can actually make the cold worse!

Fortunately, there are things to do to make colds—or any infection—a little easier to take.

If mono's got you, the best thing to do is jump into Morpheus's arms and let the body's defenses do their thing. Time and rest are the best-known cure. As for the flu, it's kind of like a hurricane. It ravages you for a few days, but when it's gone, it's gone.

But the common cold—now there's a villain you can wage war with. Mother Nature has a whole arsenal to duel it and the fatigue it brings.

Although the jury is still out on vitamin C's ability to counterpunch colds, there remain reams of evidence to stand in its defense as an offense. Some studies have even linked C to the body's production of interferon, a dynamic virus-fighting protein.

Vitamin A hasn't gotten the ink that vitamin C has, but it remains another forceful anticold trouble-shooter. Vitamin A is a vital ingredient in the body's mucus. Low levels of vitamin A, a common problem in America, mean weak mucus, which in turn weakens the first line of defense against the insidious cold viruses.

Zinc is part of the second line. Research has revealed that zinc, a major ally in the body's germ-fighting forces, may shorten colds if taken in the form of lozenges dissolved in the mouth. Vitamin B_6, pantothenate and folate are forces that boost the body's total immune defenses and help keep another disease from attacking the flanks while you're battling a cold or flu.

If you're drained, have a scratchy throat and suspect trouble on the way, tone down the night life and ask for the morning off from work. Simplify your diet. Drink a lot of fluids. If you smoke, stop or cut down. Let

Where No Cold Has Gone Before

They were called the most expensive colds in history. The Apollo 9 space mission, a dress rehearsal for the Apollo 11 moon landing, blasted off March 3, 1969—4 days late. The reason? Astronauts James McDivitt, David Scott and Russell Schweickart caught colds.

"Fatigue can be a symptom of a bad cold," explained NASA flight surgeon Walter Davis, M.D. "There exists the potential for a decrease in the ability of a person to function.

"The main concern, though, is ear blocks or sinus blocks," Dr. Davis stressed. "This is the same for people flying on commercial airliners."

the body build its forces for the coming invasion.

Heat helps, be it steam or hot towels, because viruses don't like it. They'll retreat from the nasal passages if things get steamy.

And here's a folk cure you'll love, because love's the cure! Believe it or not, a study in England determined that emotional stress—loss of a lover or a job, loneliness—increased the brawn of the heartless virus, while those who had ample friends and lovers had lighter symptoms. However, just hold off on the actual loving for a while lest you spread your viral misfortune.

Remember those house plants you chatted with back in the 1970s, when interfacing with your ficus was hip? Keep 'em around. They breathe moisture into the air, which keeps your schnozz from drying out and becoming vulnerable to a vile viral attack!

Postoperative Fatigue

Guzzling grape juice right after a tonsillectomy? Fearlessly facing eye surgery? Exercising after a gallbladder operation? Popping out of bed after an episiotomy or cesarean birth?

Sure. That's the *last* thing you can do or want to do. *Au contraire!* It's exactly what doctors prescribe to beat surgical fatigue.

"The most important aspect of recovery and fighting postoperative fatigue after a tonsillectomy is maintaining fluid intake," says Harvey Wine, M.D., of Miami, Florida. "Of course, in my field, this is a problem. People don't want to swallow because of the pain, which is understandable. This is where communication with the patient is important. I explain that the more you drink, the less it

hurts, because it moistens the throat. You'll have less long-term pain and a lot less fatigue."

"In my area, it's fear that I must overcome," says eye surgeon Merrill Knopf, M.D. of Long Beach, California. "The eyes, blindness—this really strikes a nerve. Patients who are relaxed going in heal faster and have more energy. To do this, I really try to tune in to my patients, know them personally."

General surgeon Gerald Moss, M.D., Ph.D., of Troy, New York, says getting his patients moving after surgery is essential to beating fatigue.

"The biggest complaint after surgery is, 'I tire easily.' This is, in part, because of inactivity and loss of muscle mass. That's why I have my patients walking up and down the

The Tired Zone

There's a big difference between the time it takes to completely get back on your feet after an operation and the time it takes for the normal body to heal thoroughly. The chart, which shows approximations, dramatizes this difference.

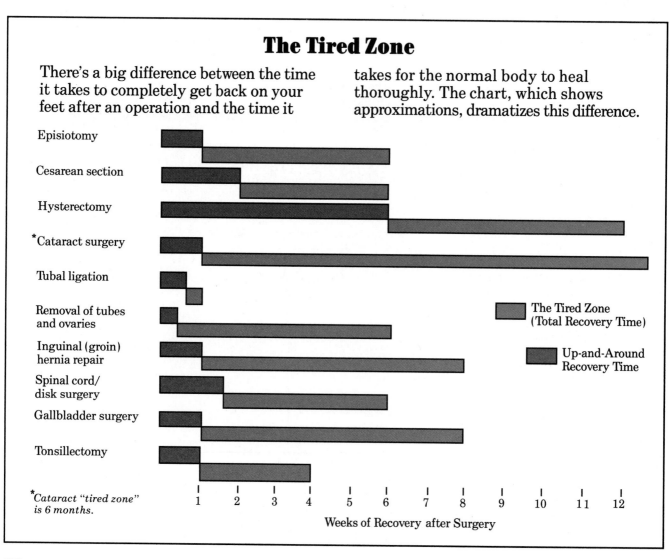

Episiotomy

Cesarean section

Hysterectomy

*Cataract surgery

Tubal ligation

Removal of tubes and ovaries

Inguinal (groin) hernia repair

Spinal cord/ disk surgery

Gallbladder surgery

Tonsillectomy

The Tired Zone (Total Recovery Time)

Up-and-Around Recovery Time

*Cataract "tired zone" is 6 months.

Weeks of Recovery after Surgery

1 2 3 4 5 6 7 8 9 10 11 12

hall within hours. Eating is also vital. What most people accept as normal, I call starvation. It takes about ten days for a surgery patient to stop breaking down protein as part of the healing process. During this period it's vital that they replace it."

Any time you cut the body, you need at least six weeks to return to a positive nitrogen balance. This imbalance is what fatigues you—you are not building as much protein as you are breaking down. The longer and more extensive the operation, the longer the recovery time.

"Technologic advances have modernized surgery and hospitalization periods have grown shorter—but the body hasn't changed!" says Dr. Knopf. "Your body still requires the same amount of time to heal—a minimum of six to eight weeks. It can take up to three weeks for the anesthesia to leave the body."

One of the best ways to beat postoperative fatigue is to go into "training" prior to the operation! Beef up the body's nutritional reserves with meat, vegetables and fruits. Stabilize your weight, dropping some if you're overweight, adding some if you're too thin. Exercise to keep the muscles strong and active and, if you smoke, try to stop *before* the operation. The reason for all this is that the body uses extra energy during the healing phase, energy that comes mostly from stored sugars. If this supply is low prior to the operation, the energy drain will tax your system.

Specifically, vitamin C is a major aid to healing because it's critical to producing the wound-healing collagen tissues the body manufactures and it helps fight infection. Vitamin A also bolsters collagen, the "cement" that holds tissue together.

The B vitamins play major roles in healing. Thiamine helps utilize carbohydrates, which provide energy and help combat fatigue. Riboflavin helps utilize protein, the raw material needed to heal wounds. Niacin aids both—carbohydrates and protein— while pantothenate insures the proper function of the adrenal glands to fight postoperative stress. Also, folate, B_{12} and riboflavin help build healthy red blood cells.

The Surgery Blues

Your body has been invaded by sharp surgical instruments. You've been cut. You've bled. You've been put into a deep, unnatural sleep. Physically, your body has undergone tremendous trauma. But that's not all. Mentally, the scars can cut as deep. The result? Fatigue. Here's help.

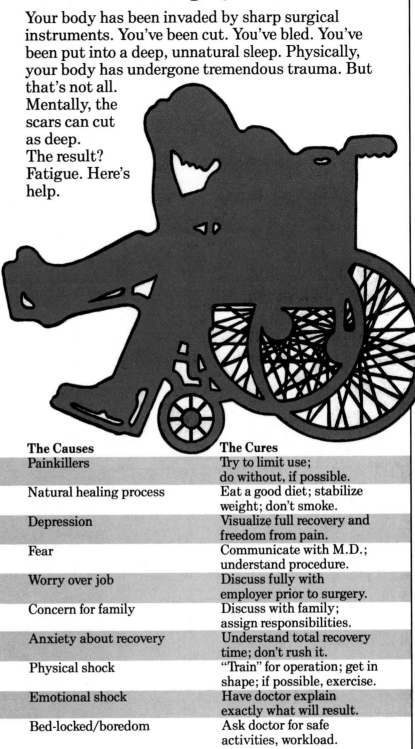

The Causes	The Cures
Painkillers	Try to limit use; do without, if possible.
Natural healing process	Eat a good diet; stabilize weight; don't smoke.
Depression	Visualize full recovery and freedom from pain.
Fear	Communicate with M.D.; understand procedure.
Worry over job	Discuss fully with employer prior to surgery.
Concern for family	Discuss with family; assign responsibilities.
Anxiety about recovery	Understand total recovery time; don't rush it.
Physical shock	"Train" for operation; get in shape; if possible, exercise.
Emotional shock	Have doctor explain exactly what will result.
Bed-locked/boredom	Ask doctor for safe activities, workload.

And don't forget the alphabetical caboose—zinc. This mineral is frequently depleted during surgery, which is double trouble because it is vital to producing the wound-healing collagen needed to repair and reenergize the body. Liver is a top source of both B vitamins *and* zinc.

Thyroid Problems

In an episode of the classic television series "Star Trek," Captain Kirk was slipped a "Mickey" of Scalosian water, a substance that put rocket fuel in his metabolic system. Kirk's body was revved so high he became "invisible" to his crewmates. Dr. "Bones" McCoy and science officer Spock astutely determined that Kirk had mankind's worst case of hyperthyroidism—too much thyroid hormone in the system. They cured him, of course, and in the process were able to repel an invasion of hyperthyroid aliens who were trying to capture the ship. Medical science (fiction) prevails!

It was an exciting yarn, one that vividly demonstrates the power and function of the thyroid gland.

In terms of fatigue, it's the reverse of Captain Kirk's dilemma that haunts Earthlings. If the thyroid slacks off and doesn't produce enough of the vital energy hormone thyroxine, hypothyroidism results.

Hypothyroid individuals are always tired, says Isadore Rosenfeld, M.D., author of *The Second Opinion*. They tend to sleep a great deal. The voice is hoarse and low pitched. The speech is slow. They are less alert, often hard of hearing. "They are also often depressed, and for good reason. Life isn't much fun," he says.

Chronic fatigue is a major result of hypothyroidism. Weight gain, sensitivity to cold temperatures, dry skin and hair loss are other symptoms that take the fun out of life.

A Giant's Sad Story

Wilt "The Stilt" Chamberlain. Akeem "The Dream" Olajuwon. Ed "Too Tall" Jones. Robert "too tall" Wadlow. Robert who?

At 8′ 11″, Wadlow was nearly 2 feet taller than today's stratospheric athletes. Unlike them, his height wasn't attributed to good genes and nutrition. He soared to the greatest height in recorded history due to a malfunction of his pituitary, a growth gland which helps to regulate the thyroid.

Instead of being dubbed a "superstar," Wadlow is described in medical terms: a victim of gigantism and acromegaly. Instead of executing leaping slam dunks and blocked kicks, he needed supports to walk. His coordination was poor, his strength minimal, and his life short. He died in 1940 at the age of 22 due to cellulitis, a minor infection caused by his leg braces.

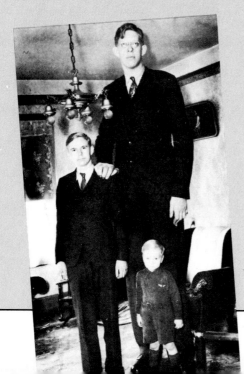

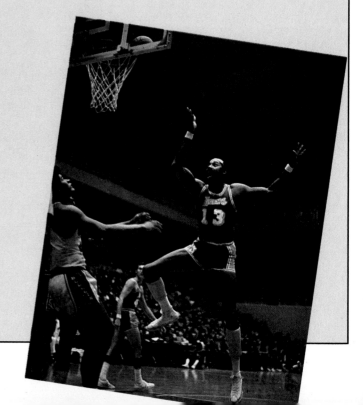

Hypothyroidism, like anemia, circulatory problems, diabetes and allergies, can tap your energy without revealing itself. In fact, it's difficult to detect even after extensive tests.

Mild cases often register "normal" in lab tests. This is because what may be normal levels of thyroid hormones for one person are low levels for another. Allow this "low" to linger for a few years and other fatigue-complicating problems can arise, including anemia, high blood cholesterol, slow heart rate and slow reflexes.

TUNE UP THE TIRED THYROID

Dr. McCoy's quick discovery and remedy for Captain Kirk's trouble was not the result of futuristic medical advances, or even of imaginative script writers. Even today thyroid trouble is treatable. The value of the treatments is demonstrated by professional football player Ed Newman. The massive, muscular athlete has anchored the Miami Dolphin offensive line for ten years—and he doesn't even have a thyroid gland! It was surgically removed after cancer struck. Newman has been able to excel at a sport where energy is paramount because thyroid drugs have replaced the natural function of the missing gland. In the same manner, lower doses can boost a weak gland, providing the precise chemical balance for peak energy.

There are cautions. Thyroid drugs, if taken unnecessarily or in high doses, can make you nervous and irritable, promote a rapid, irregular heartbeat and induce weight loss (they are *not* to be used for weight control, however). In addition, radioactive-iodine therapy or surgery to treat hyperthyroidism can slow down the thyroid too much, producing the fatigue and other symptoms of a sluggish thyroid.

Nature provides additional ways to cheer up a depressed thyroid. Iodine is needed to produce the thyroid's energy hormone. Without it, the thyroid swells in an attempt to maintain production. Often it still comes up short. The ensuing goiter

Cure My Wife—Please!

Here's a twist to an old saying—"hypothyroid victims of a feather, doze through life together." That's what thyroid therapy pioneer Broda O. Barnes, M.D., discovered when he cured an unhealthy thyroid and in turn nearly ruined a healthy marriage.

Dr. Barnes tells of a man who came into his office one day, grossly overweight and suffering from deep fatigue. He could barely get through a day's work. Dr. Barnes's prescription—thyroid therapy and diet control. It worked.

Unfortunately, the man's wife wasn't as pleased as Dr. Barnes. Her new pepperpot husband was not what she bargained for when she said "I do." The man returned to Dr. Barnes, saying the marriage was shot, referring to his wife as "tired, cross, unwilling to go out at night." Dr. Barnes, realizing that hypothyroids tend to marry other hypothyroids, had the answer. "Nature had thrown them together. If they were to enjoy life, I would have to treat her, also. Her husband brought her in, I gave her the same treatment and it worked. Like in the story books, 'they lived happily ever after!'"

can grow so large it compresses the throat. To avoid these unpleasantries, iodized salt has been introduced into the world diet. However, salt may boost blood pressure in people who are prone to that problem. If you're on a salt-free diet, look toward the sea. Fish is a good source of iodine; haddock, cod, shrimp, sea perch, halibut, herring, mackerel, sardines, bluefish and sea bass are particularly iodine rich.

If you're being treated for hypothyroidism, you might want to watch your vitamin E intake. In one study, vitamin E caused a significant reduction of thyroid hormone. The counterpunch affects only certain individuals (woman on oral contraceptives seem to be exempt), and it is possible that vitamin E reduces the level of thyroid hormone required by mimicking its action. Consult your doctor.

Hypothyroidism in infants, a problem associated with mental retardation, may be tempered by breast feeding. This is because mother's milk contains a significantly higher amount of thyroid hormone than cow's milk or popular formulas.

Source Notes

Chapter 1
Page 5

"Who Are the Stress Seekers?" based on material from *Life Stress*, by Rosalind Forbes, Ed.D. (New York: Doubleday & Co., 1979).

Chapter 2
Page 28

"High-Fat Foods" adapted from *Nutritive Value of American Foods in Common Units*, Agriculture Handbook No. 456, by Catherine F. Adams (Washington, D.C.: Agricultural Research Service, U.S. Department of Agriculture, 1975) and *Composition of Foods: Fats and Oils*, Agriculture Handbook No. 8-4, by Consumer and Food Economics Institute (Washington, D.C.: Science and Education Administration, U.S. Department of Agriculture, 1979) and *Composition of Foods: Dairy and Egg Products*, Agriculture Handbook No. 8-1, by Consumer and Food Economics Institute (Washington, D.C.: Agricultural Research Service, U.S. Department of Agriculture, 1976) and *Composition of Foods: Sausages and Luncheon Meats*, Agriculture Handbook No. 8-7, by Consumer Nutrition Center (Washington, D.C.: Science and Education Administration, U.S. Department of Agriculture, 1980) and *Composition of Foods: Fruits and Fruit Juices*, Agriculture Handbook No. 8-9, by Consumer Nutrition Center (Washington, D.C.: Human Nutrition Information Service, U.S. Department of Agriculture, 1982) and *Proximate Composition of Beef from Carcass to Cooked Meat: Method of Derivation and Tables of Values*, Home Economics Research Report No. 31, by Consumer and Food Economics Division (Washington, D.C.: Agricultural Research Service, U.S. Department of Agriculture, 1972).

Page 29

"Low-Fat Foods" adapted from *Nutritive Value of American Foods in Common Units*, Agriculture Handbook No. 456, by Catherine F. Adams (Washington, D.C.: Agricultural Research Service, U.S. Department of Agriculture, 1975) and *Composition of Foods: Fruits and Fruit Juices*, Agriculture Handbook No. 8-9, by Consumer Nutrition Center (Washington, D.C.: Human Nutrition Information Service, U.S. Department of Agriculture, 1982) and *Composition of Foods: Breakfast Cereals*, Agriculture Handbook No. 8-8, by Consumer Nutrition Center (Washington, D.C.: Human Nutrition Information Service, U.S. Department of Agriculture, 1982) and *Composition of Foods: Dairy and Egg Products*, Agriculture Handbook No. 8-1, by Consumer and Food Economics Institute (Washington, D.C.: Agricultural Research Service, U.S. Department of Agriculture, 1976) and *Composition of Foods: Poultry Products*, Agriculture Handbook No. 8-5, by Consumer and Food Economics Institute (Washington, D.C.: Science and Education Administration, U.S. Department of Agriculture, 1979) and *Composition of Foods: Soups, Sauces and Gravies*, Agriculture Handbook No. 8-6, by Consumer and Food Economics Institute (Washington, D.C.: Science and Education Administration, U.S. Department of Agriculture, 1980) and *Proximate Composition of Beef from Carcass to Cooked Meat: Method of Derivation and Tables of Values*, Home Economics Research Report No. 31, by Consumer and Food Economics Division (Washington, D.C.: Agricultural Research Service, U.S. Department of Agriculture, 1972).

Chapter 6
Page 82

"The No-Jet-Lag Diet" created by Charles Ehret, Ph.D., of the U.S. Department of Energy's Argonne National Laboratory.

Chapter 9
Page 134

"Test Your Sensitivity; Are You Weather Sensitive?" adapted from *Weathering* by Stephen Rosen. Copyright 1979 by Stephen Rosen. Reprinted by permission of the publisher, M. Evans and Co., Inc., New York, New York 10017.

Chapter 11
Page 153

"High Fiber Equals High Energy" compiled from information provided by Nutrient Data Research Group, U.S. Department of Agriculture.

Photography Credits

Cover: Margaret Skrovanek.
Staff Photographers— Angelo M. Caggiano: pp. 109; 136-137. Carl Doney: pp. 60-61; 76-77; 79; 114; 115, bottom; 142-143. T. L. Gettings: pp. 93, 102-103; 105; 115, top; 146, top left and bottom right. John P. Hamel: pp. 16-17; 48; 86-87; 90; 111; 146, bottom left. Donna Hornberger: p. 23. Mark Lenny: p. 140. Mitchell T. Mandel: pp. 24; 32-33. Alison Miksch: pp. 19; 22-23; 72-73. Scott Schmidt: pp. 94-95. Margaret Skrovanek: pp. 37; 44-45; 51; 53; 108; 124; 127; 129. Christie C. Tito: pp. 40-41; 85; 104; 132. Sally Shenk Ullman: pp. 34-35.

Other Photographers— David Epperson: pp. 56-57. Armando Gallo/ Shooting Star: p. 6, right. Gates/Frederic Lewis, Inc.: p. 152 (Mary Tyler Moore, Minnie Pearl, H. G. Wells). Bob Griffith: p. 146, top right. John Iacono/*Sports Illustrated:* pp. 144-145. Yoram Kahana©/Shooting Star: p. 152 (Menachem Begin). Richard Laird/Leo de Wys, Inc.: p. 47. Lambert/ Frederic Lewis, Inc.: pp. 12, bottom; 119. David Madison© 1984/Duomo: p. 7, top. Kurt Muller/ Doubleday and Co., Inc.: p. 7, left. Barry Parker/ Bruce Coleman, Inc.: pp. 116-117. John Severson/ *Wind Surf* magazine: pp. viii-1. Charles Steiner/ Picture Group Photo: p. 13, top. Tony Triolo/*Sports Illustrated:* p. 8, right. Jerry Wachter/Focus on Sports, Inc.: pp. 152 (Bobby Jones); 160, right. Charles Weckler© 1983/ The Image Bank: p. 68, left.

*Additional Photographs Courtesy of—*AP/World Wide Photos: p. 8, left. Auroratone Foundation of America, Inc., Hollywood: p. 131. Robert Caputo Photography: p. 13, bottom. Leo de Wys, Inc.: p. 9, right. Devaney Stock Photos: pp. 12, left; 152 (Ty Cobb, Thomas Edison, Jackie Robinson). Focus on Sports, Inc.: pp. 7, bottom; 39; 152 (Bobby Clark). *The Guinness Book of World Records*, Sterling Publishing Co., Inc., © 1984, Guinness Superlatives, Ltd.: p. 160, left. Claudia Kunin Photography: p. 9, left. Frederic Lewis, Inc.: p. 152 (Jack Benny, Ernest Hemingway, Howard Hughes, Spencer Tracy). National Aeronautics and Space Administration: p. 156. Lee Perry of Samadhi Tank Co., Los Angeles: p. 106. Philadelphia Museum of Art, Mr. and Mrs. Carroll S. Tyson Collection: p. 68, right. Shostal Associates: p. 152 (Nikita Khrushchev).

Index

Photographic Styling Credits

Barbara Fritz: p. 19.
Donna Hornberger: pp.
136-137. Kurt Swinehart:
pp. 72-73; 136-137. J. C.
Vera: pp. 108; 124;
136-137.

Illustration Credits

Bascove: pp. 4; 67; 83;
89; 97. Susan Gray: pp.
63; 113; 123; 139; 147;
151; 153. Irene Hecht: p.
6, left. Mary Anne Shea:
pp. 3; 12-13; 40-41; 65;
80-81; 112; 126; 130;
148-149; 154-155; 159.
Elwood Smith: pp. 25,
54; 88; 91; 98-99; 107;
125. Chris Spollen: pp.
8-9; 62; 82; 120.

Recipe Development

Judith Benn Hurley,
Nancy J. Zelko

Special Thanks to—
Fisher-Price, East Aurora,
N.Y.; Parkette National
Gymnastic Training
Center, Allentown, Pa.

Rodale Press, Inc., publishes PREVENTION®, the better health magazine.
For information on how to order your subscription,
write to PREVENTION®, Emmaus, PA 18049.